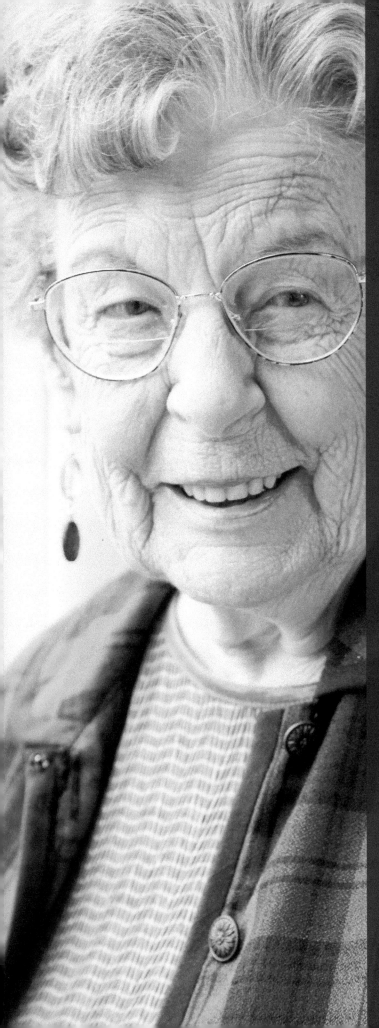

Nursing Older People

at a Glance

Edited by

Josie Tetley

Nigel Cox

Kirsten Jack

Gary Witham

all at

The Faculty of Health,
Psychology and Social Care
Manchester Metropolitan University
Manchester, UK

Series Editor: Ian Peate OBE, FRCN

WILEY Blackwell

Registered Offices: John Wiley & Sons, Inc., 111 River Street, Hoboken, NJ 07030, USA
John Wiley & Sons, Ltd., The Atrium, Southern Gate, Chichester, West Sussex, PO19 8SQ, UK

Editorial Office: 9600 Garsington Road, Oxford, OX4 2DQ, UK

For details of our global editorial offices, customer services, and more information about Wiley products visit us at www.wiley.com.

Library of Congress Cataloging-in-Publication Data are available

ISBN: 9781119043867

Cover image: © FangXiaNuo/Shutterstock
Cover design by Wiley

Set in Minion Pro 9.5/11.5 pt by Aptara

10 9 8 7 6 5 4 3 2 1

Contents

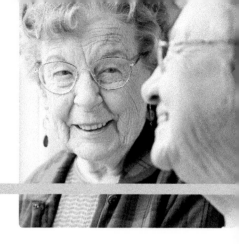

Contributors

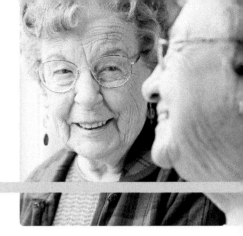

Razia Aubdool, Chapters 16 and 17

Canan Birimoğlu, Chapter 15

Louise Bowden, Chapters 16 and 17

Jacqueline M. Cash, Chapter 10

Michelle Croston, Chapter 3

Nigel Cox, Chapters 24 and 38

Donna Davenport, Chapter 25

Jan Dewing, Chapter 26

Garry Diack, Chapter 36

Fiona Duncan, Chapter 8

Chris Ellis, Chapter 9

Marilyn Fitzpatrick, Chapter 41

David Garbutt, Chapter 29

Linda Garbutt, Chapter 2

Robin Hadley, Chapter 34

Carol Haigh, Chapter 8

Caroline Holland, Chapter 43

Maxine Holt, Chapter 14

Lindesay Irvine, Chapters 18, 20 and 39

Kirsten Jack, Chapters 4, 21, 38 and 45

Emma-Reetta Koivunen, Chapters 42 and 44

Janet Marsden, Chapter 7

Jamie McPhee, Chapter 22

Julie Messenger, Chapter 6

Eula Miller, Chapters 27 and 31

Duncan Mitchell, Chapter 36

Gayatri Nambiar-Greenwood, Chapters 1 and 32

Stewart Rickels, Chapters 19 and 40

Caroline Ridley, Chapter 30

Stuart Roberts, Chapter 35

Carol Rushton, Chapter 25

Clare Street, Chapter 5

Stuart Taylor, Introduction

Josie Tetley, Chapters 21, 24, 42 and 45

Lucy Webb, Chapter 37

Danita Wilmott, Chapter 12

Gary Witham, Chapters 11, 13, 23, 28 and 33

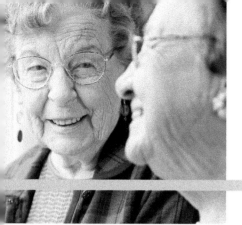

Introduction

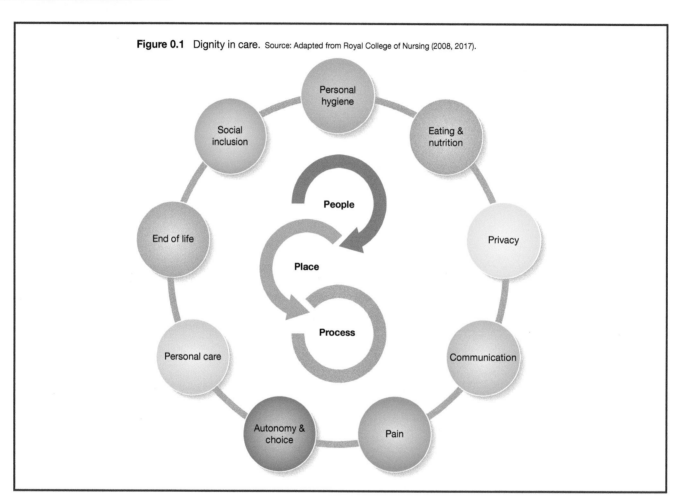

Figure 0.1 Dignity in care. Source: Adapted from Royal College of Nursing (2008, 2017).

Our aims for this book

This book is primarily aimed at undergraduate and post-qualification nurses who care for older people in a range of care settings including hospital, community, residential and other health or social care settings. The editors and contributing authors believe that this book will also be of value to a wide range of practitioners working in a nursing or a nurse-related capacity, for instance pre-registration nurses, healthcare assistants, associate practitioners, registered nurses working in both the NHS and independent care home sectors, and those returning to a career in nursing.

Nurses are under increasing pressure to demonstrate that the care they deliver is supported by best evidence, compassionate and person-centred. For nurses working with older people this can be challenging, as people's needs in later life are often complex and diverse. This book therefore provides an accessible overview of key concepts that can help nurses understand how care in practice can be more person-centred, while also promoting dignity, health and well-being.

How the book is organised

The book is divided into six parts. Part 1 introduces concepts central to dignified and compassionate person-centred care. Part 2 explores health and well-being, including essential aspects of living such as sleep, the senses and nutrition. Part 3 focuses

Nursing Older People at a Glance, First Edition. Edited by Josie Tetley, Nigel Cox, Kirsten Jack and Gary Witham.
© 2018 John Wiley & Sons, Ltd. Published 2018 by John Wiley & Sons, Ltd.

upon health promotion, and incorporates a diverse range of topics including physical activity and the arts. Parts 4 and 5 address complexity and diversity in older people's care, including topics such as mental well-being, diverse communities and learning disability. Part 6 concludes the book, and illustrates how environments of care impact on practice. Autonomy and independence are central principles, and the role of assistive technologies and the challenges of working with older people in a diverse range of contexts are considered.

Dignity as a core concept for older people's care

Dignity in care work focuses on the value of every person as an individual. It means respecting others' views, choices and decisions, not making assumptions about how people want to be treated and working with care and compassion

Skills for Care, 2017

The concept of dignity shapes all of the chapters in this book. However, making dignity in care a reality also means that nurses and other healthcare professionals need to be able to understand what this means in the context of people, places and processes in multiple and complex ways (Figure 0.1). The importance of dignity in care is also underpinned by the Nursing and Midwifery Council (NMC) code of conduct (Figure 0.2) which, at the time of writing, states that nurses must:

Figure 0.2 The Nursing Midwifery Council (NMC) code of conduct. Source: Nursing & Midwifery Council (2015).

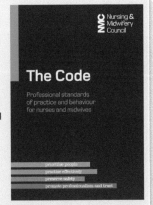

1 Treat people as individuals and uphold their dignity.
To achieve this you must:
1.1 Treat people with kindness, respect and compassion.
1.2 Make sure you deliver the fundamentals of care effectively.
1.3 Avoid making assumptions and recognise diversity and individual choice.
1.4 Make sure that any treatment, assistance or care for which you are responsible is delivered without undue delay, and
1.5 Respect and uphold people's rights.

When considering dignity-related matters for patients we tend to think of some of the more personal situations such as receiving assistance with bathing, dressing or toileting, but recommendations from Age UK (2013) serve to remind nurses of the need to think widely and creatively about older people's care. From admission to hospital or any point of care, it is important to develop a professional but caring relationship that takes account of the wider and more holistic needs of older people and their carers. This book provides some practical guidance about how these needs can be met in ways that uphold dignity in care. However, it is also important to remember that understanding and appreciating individual values, beliefs and practices is not easy, and key areas related to dignity need to be considered from the outset of the patient journey (Royal College of Nursing, 2008, 2017); again, key chapters in this book provide guidance about good practice in nursing on this.

The editors and authors who have contributed to the development of this book recognise that there are no easy solutions to providing individualised and dignified care for older people. By providing a range of short, but succinct evidence-based chapters, this book presents guidance about key concepts that can support dignity in care in the context of the key difficulties and challenges that nurses encounter in practice.

Josie Tetley
Nigel Cox
Kirsten Jack
Gary Witham
Stuart Taylor

References

Age UK (2103) Delivering Dignity: Securing dignity in care for older people in hospitals and care homes. London: Age UK. Available at: http://www.ageuk.org.uk/Global/Delivering%20Dignity%20Report.pdf?dtrk=true (accessed 27 September 2017).

Nursing and Midwifery Council (2015) The Code. Professional standards of practice and behaviour for nurses and midwives. London: NMC. Available at: https://www.nmc.org.uk/globalassets/sitedocuments/nmc-publications/nmc-code.pdf (accessed 27 September 2017).

Royal College of Nursing (2008) Dignity at the heart of everything we do: Defending Dignity – Challenges and opportunities for nursing. London: Royal College of Nursing. Available at: http://www.dignityincare.org.uk/_assets/RCN_Digntiy_at_the_heart_of_everything_we_do.pdf (accessed 27 September 2017).

Royal College of Nursing (2017) Preserving people's dignity. First steps for health care assistants. London: Royal College of Nursing. Available at: http://rcnhca.org.uk/equality-diversity-and-rights/preserving-peoples-dignity/ (accessed 27 September 2017).

Skills for Care (2017) Dignity in care work. Leeds/London: Skills for Care. Available at: http://www.skillsforcare.org.uk/Topics/Dignity/Dignity.aspx (accessed 27 September 2017).

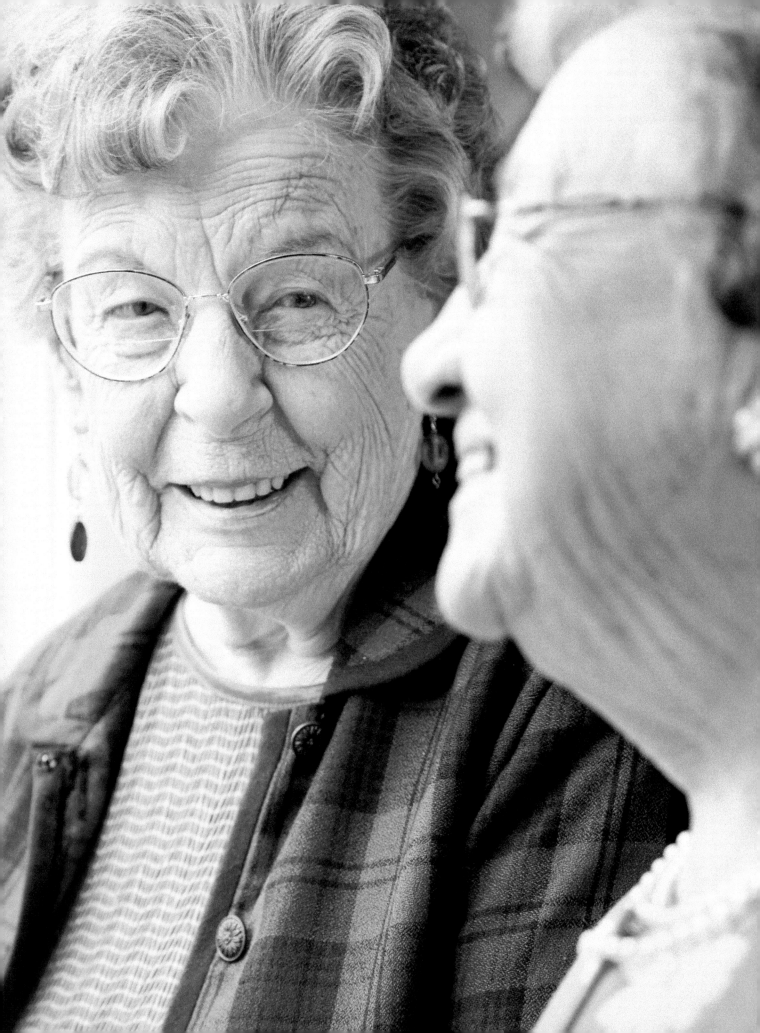

Person-centred care in practice

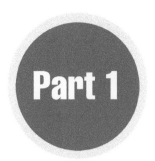

Part 1

Chapters

1 Promoting person-centred care

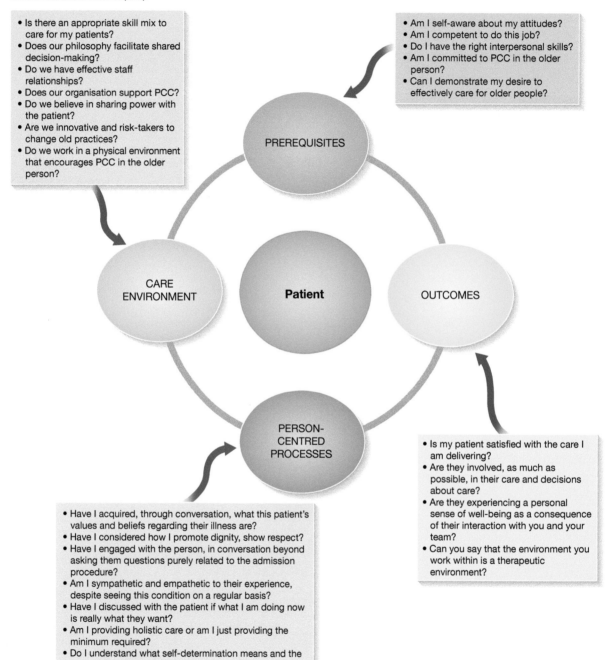

Figure 1.1 Adaptation of the McCormack and McCance constructs for Person-Centred Nursing Framework. Source: Adapted from McCormack and McCance (2010).

- Is there an appropriate skill mix to care for my patients?
- Does our philosophy facilitate shared decision-making?
- Do we have effective staff relationships?
- Does our organisation support PCC?
- Do we believe in sharing power with the patient?
- Are we innovative and risk-takers to change old practices?
- Do we work in a physical environment that encourages PCC in the older person?

- Am I self-aware about my attitudes?
- Am I competent to do this job?
- Do I have the right interpersonal skills?
- Am I committed to PCC in the older person?
- Can I demonstrate my desire to effectively care for older people?

PREREQUISITES

CARE ENVIRONMENT

Patient

OUTCOMES

PERSON-CENTRED PROCESSES

- Is my patient satisfied with the care I am delivering?
- Are they involved, as much as possible, in their care and decisions about care?
- Are they experiencing a personal sense of well-being as a consequence of their interaction with you and your team?
- Can you say that the environment you work within is a therapeutic environment?

- Have I acquired, through conversation, what this patient's values and beliefs regarding their illness are?
- Have I considered how I promote dignity, show respect?
- Have I engaged with the person, in conversation beyond asking them questions purely related to the admission procedure?
- Am I sympathetic and empathetic to their experience, despite seeing this condition on a regular basis?
- Have I discussed with the patient if what I am doing now is really what they want?
- Am I providing holistic care or am I just providing the minimum required?
- Do I understand what self-determination means and the concept of purposeful living?

To provide person-centred care (PCC) for any patient or client means that they are included in decision making about their care. PCC in the older person cannot be successful unless the ethos of the wider MDT is one of a shared partnership with each other and the patient.

In order for PCC to be effective for all concerned, nurses involved in caring for the older person need to be aware of a number of factors. This involves not only looking at the needs of the patient and considering their definition of satisfaction, but also, fundamentally, staff considering their understanding of older people and PCC itself.

It is important that nurses have an awareness of their own attitudes regarding older people. The media often portrays older people as being dependant on others and it is inevitable that this will have an unconscious effect on our attitude (Koskinen *et al.*, 2014) and affect our interpersonal skills that are fundamental to effective PCC. In not acknowledging the diversity of the older population, in terms of their ability and capacity, we are reducing them to a homogeneous group incapable of being asked about or making decisions of their own, for themselves (Phelan, 2011). By becoming aware of culturally influenced attitudes about the older person and how these outlooks are mirrored in the ways older people are observed, treated and cared for in society, the nurse and the MDT can better understand the premise from which to provide high-quality PCC.

McCormack and McCance (2010) developed a 'Person-Centred Nursing Framework' and this framework has four constructs that are fundamental to delivering PCC in the older person effectively. They are:

- Prerequisites
- The care environment
- Person-centred processes
- Outcomes.

These constructs are presented in Figure 1.1 with examples of the questions the nurse might consider when delivering PCC in the older person.

Having taken into consideration the constructs above as fundamental to delivering effective PCC, the nurse, due to cultural differences, also needs to appreciate those intrinsic factors that will affect what can be called the 'intergenerational conversation' that occurs between the patient and nurse.

Bochner (2013) asserted that intersubjective values such as power, hierarchy, status, subordination and perceptions of equality affect intergenerational conversation more than previously imagined. Bochner emphasises that any contact between professional and patient can affect the communication and behaviour of both parties due to the interaction being a heavily differing value-oriented encounter. Intergenerational communication does not just include the entire range of communication skills across boundaries of age groups but also takes into account gender and cultural factors.

An awareness of these factors is important if the patient is going to be comfortable to express their needs and for the nurse–patient relationship to be mutually beneficial. It is important for the nurse to be aware of the intergenerational implications of both verbal and non-verbal aspects of conversing with those who are of a different age group, and perhaps, feeling vulnerable in a care setting. As mentioned at the beginning of this chapter, it is essential that the nurse be aware of his or her own socialised prejudices or prejudgements that may affect their interpersonal behaviour. Both these traits affect the tone and values of conversation that follows, in which the patient comes to recognise the identity that the nurse is now giving them, be it positively or negatively (Samovar *et al.*, 2013).

The notion of PCC is complex and multi-dimensional. For it to be successful, the MDT needs to work at sustaining a reflective and honest planned culture change, which is necessary to embed the values of PCC of older people in daily practices. Good nurse leadership and the care environment are key influencing factors on the way that person-centredness is experienced by patients, their families and the MDT. For PCC to be experienced in a consistent and continuous way by these patients, the culture of practice has to support a compassionate, humanistic and creative way of practising, that enables care teams to flourish or achieve patient satisfaction. In adopting this change in culture, ultimately, the nurse is working towards promoting those notions around self-determination and purposeful living, often taken for granted when we are young.

References

Bochner, S. (2013) *Cultures in Contact: Studies in Cross-Cultural Interaction*. Oxford: Pergamon Press.

Koskinen, S., Salminen, L. and Leino-Kilpi, H. (2014) Media portrayal of older people as illustrated in Finnish newspapers. *International Journal of Qualitative Studies on Health and Well-being*. doi: 10.3402/qhw.v9.25304.

McCormack, B. and McCance, T. (2010) *Person-Centred Nursing: Theory, Models and Methods*. Oxford: Blackwell Publishing.

Phelan, A. (2011) Socially constructing older people: Examining discourses which can shape nurses' understanding and practice. *Journal of Advanced Nursing* 67: 893–903.

Samovar, L.A., Porter, R.E. and McDaniel, E.R. (2013) *Intercultural Communication: A Reader*, 11th edn. London: Thompson Learning.

2 Capacity and consent

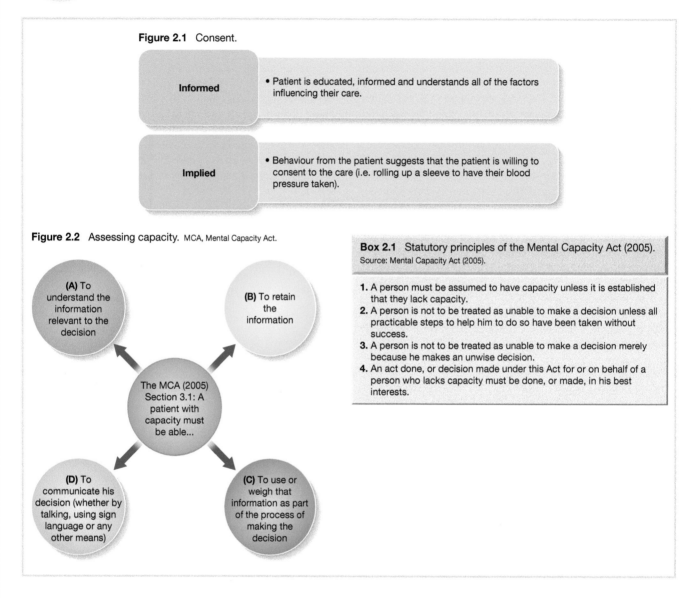

Figure 2.1 Consent.

| Informed | • Patient is educated, informed and understands all of the factors influencing their care. |

| Implied | • Behaviour from the patient suggests that the patient is willing to consent to the care (i.e. rolling up a sleeve to have their blood pressure taken). |

Figure 2.2 Assessing capacity. MCA, Mental Capacity Act.

The MCA (2005) Section 3.1: A patient with capacity must be able...

(A) To understand the information relevant to the decision

(B) To retain the information

(C) To use or weigh that information as part of the process of making the decision

(D) To communicate his decision (whether by talking, using sign language or any other means)

Box 2.1 Statutory principles of the Mental Capacity Act (2005). Source: Mental Capacity Act (2005).

1. A person must be assumed to have capacity unless it is established that they lack capacity.
2. A person is not to be treated as unable to make a decision unless all practicable steps to help him to do so have been taken without success.
3. A person is not to be treated as unable to make a decision merely because he makes an unwise decision.
4. An act done, or decision made under this Act for or on behalf of a person who lacks capacity must be done, or made, in his best interests.

Consent is one of the cornerstones of good healthcare practice. It enables patients to exercise their autonomy, their choices, their free will and self-determination. Patients should no longer feel passive recipients of care, rather consumers of a health service where equity, respect and mutuality are recognised (Department of Health, 2012). The promotion of consent allows practitioners to develop therapeutic relationships with patients and service users, promoting reciprocity, equality and trust, all of which are fundamental to the core values within the National Health Service Constitution (Department of Health, 2015). Thus, all individuals receiving care, where possible, must give their permission for that care to be delivered.

Consent

Conceptually, consent can be divided into two distinct categories: informed and implied consent (Figure 2.1).

The Nursing and Midwifery Council (2015) and the General Medical Council (2008) clearly articulate that any decision made by patients surrounding any aspect of their care, should be informed in nature. This requires that patients are fully aware of the reasons for their treatment, any side effects that may occur and the risk of any potential harm that may be suffered as a result of this care. Having considered all of this information, the benefits, risks and burdens, patients have the right to agree to or refuse treatment. Sometimes the refusal of treatment may be

Nursing Older People at a Glance, First Edition. Edited by Josie Tetley, Nigel Cox, Kirsten Jack and Gary Witham.
© 2018 John Wiley & Sons, Ltd. Published 2018 by John Wiley & Sons, Ltd.

seen as an unwise decision, which is detrimental to the patient's health and against the advice of the healthcare professionals; this refusal must still be respected in the competent patient (Nursing and Midwifery Council, 2015).

Informed consent needs to be integrated into all aspects of nursing care delivery, not just major surgery or medical procedures. This means that everything from assisting a patient with personal hygiene needs, to the administration of medication or the delivery of nursing procedures must be fully explained to the patient, who then agrees to the provision of that care. However, studies have suggested that informed consent prior to the delivery of nursing care is 'under-developed', with many nurses relying on implied consent and failing to respect refusal of treatment prior to the delivery of nursing procedures (Cole, 2012).

Within the context of healthcare the Professional Regulatory Bodies (General Medical Council, 2008; Nursing and Midwifery Council, 2015), statute (Mental Capacity Act 2005, Human Rights Act 1998, Criminal Justice Act 1988) and ethical practice (Nursing and Midwifery Council, 2015) drive the need for informed consent. Failure to obtain informed consent has multiple consequences; for patients their human rights are violated and the acceptable standard of care expected is compromised. For the practitioners involved, lack of adherence may lead to professional misconduct hearings, employment tribunal or liability in negligence (General Medical Council, 2008; Nursing and Midwifery Council, 2015). Furthermore, if treatment or care is provided without the patient's informed consent, civil or criminal proceedings may be instigated due to charges of battery (trespass to the person) or assault (where malicious criminal intent is proven).

Factors influencing informed consent

There are many factors that may impact upon the ability to gain informed consent from a patient, particularly if they are older. There is a need to recognise and acknowledge the diversity of the older patient population in relation to information giving and consent, thus tailoring information based around patients' individualised needs. Language, sensory impairment, literacy and cognition are all features that could influence comprehension. Nurses must take all practicable actions to facilitate understanding where possible. Therefore, providing adequate time, a quiet environment, written information in a suitable font size and the involvement of family and friends (with consent) so more people can retain the information are practical ways to facilitate this.

The Mental Capacity Act (2005)

The Mental Capacity Act (2005) (MCA) provides clear legal parameters for practitioners to promote autonomy, with the assumption that everyone (over the age of 16) has the capacity to make decisions surrounding their care unless evidence suggests otherwise (Box 2.1).

The principles given in Box 2.1 reduce the potential for paternalism and prejudice, clearly highlighting that assumptions regarding capacity should not be made purely on the basis of age, medical condition or diagnosis. Based upon this framework, it is important to note that some patients may be able to provide informed consent and refusal regarding certain aspects of their care, such as whether they wish to receive personal care; however, they may not be deemed competent to make more complex healthcare decisions.

If an individual is assessed as lacking capacity to make a decision about their care autonomously, those making a decision on their behalf must adopt the principle of 'best interest', according to the Mental Capacity Act (2005). Healthcare staff should therefore make every effort to understand what the patient would have wanted were they able to autonomously make the decision themselves. This requires the holistic assessment and understanding of the unique nature of that patient, and may require discussions with family members to establish, if not documented within an advanced decision, the wants and wishes of the patient when they had capacity.

A key issue, which must be addressed, is that family members are not able to consent on behalf of their loved one, unless they have been nominated by a Lasting Power of Attorney (LPA). Under the Mental Capacity Act, the attorney is an individual that the patient nominates to make choices about their health, welfare and the management of property, when capacity is lost. There is an official process to be followed in adopting this role and the LPA must be registered with the Office of Public Guardian.

Safeguarding the rights of those who have lost capacity is inherent within the Mental Capacity Act. Major decisions surrounding the deprivation of liberties, the instigation or withdrawal of serious medical treatment, long-term continuing care and rehousing will often require liaison with local authorities, Independent Mental Capacity Advocates (IMCAs) or court-appointed Deputies. The Court of Protection will hear cases surrounding serious medical treatment decisions and will try to resolve disputes surrounding differences of opinion between the patient's carer and healthcare workers.

In order for consent to be valid, it must be made voluntarily, without coercion, and must be provided by a mentally competent patient (see Figure 2.2).

Lack of capacity may be transient or due to a long-term health breakdown such as brain injury, mental illness, levels of consciousness, phobias, confusion, delirium, intoxication and intellectual disability.

In order to facilitate truly informed consent for the competent patient, nurses must understand the dynamics of decision-making and capacity. In reviewing the concept of competence, the transient nature of lack of capacity must be acknowledged and the notion of best interest fully understood. With this comes the need to develop and enhance effective communication, individualised holistic care and the discouragement of discrimination, deceit and coercion, enabling patients to be true partners in their care.

References

Cole, C. (2012) Implied consent and nursing practice; ethical or convenient? *Nursing Ethics* 19: 550–557.

Criminal Justice Act (1988) https://www.legislation.gov.uk/ukpga/1988/33. London: HMSO.

Department of Health (2012) Liberating the NHS; No decision about me, without me. London: HMSO.

Department of Health (2015) The NHS Constitution: the NHS belongs to us all. London: HMSO.

General Medical Council (2008) Consent: Doctors and patients making decision together. London: GMC.

Human Rights Act (1998) Available at: https://www.legislation.gov.uk/ukpga/1998/42. London: HMSO.

Mental Capacity Act (2005) Available at: http://www.legislation.gov.uk/ukpga/2005/9/contents. London: HMSO.

Nursing and Midwifery Council (2015) *The Code of Professional Standards of Practice and Behaviour for Nurses and Midwives.* London: NMC.

3 Communication

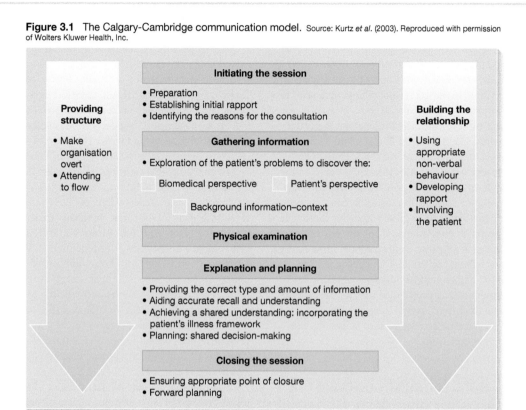

Figure 3.1 The Calgary-Cambridge communication model. Source: Kurtz *et al.* (2003). Reproduced with permission of Wolters Kluwer Health, Inc.

Providing structure

- Make organisation overt
- Attending to flow

Initiating the session

- Preparation
- Establishing initial rapport
- Identifying the reasons for the consultation

Gathering information

- Exploration of the patient's problems to discover the:

  Biomedical perspective   Patient's perspective

  Background information–context

Physical examination

Explanation and planning

- Providing the correct type and amount of information
- Aiding accurate recall and understanding
- Achieving a shared understanding: incorporating the patient's illness framework
- Planning: shared decision-making

Closing the session

- Ensuring appropriate point of closure
- Forward planning

Building the relationship

- Using appropriate non-verbal behaviour
- Developing rapport
- Involving the patient

Effective communication is critical to the health and well-being of older adults. Patients in all settings give high priority to communication as a key aspect of care, wanting above all to be treated with humanity, dignity and respect. Understanding supportive communication strategies is therefore important as these enable healthcare professionals to develop person-centred relationships, particularly with older adults. For patients, effective communication enables them to be listened to, involved in their own care and to choose between different treatment options, which facilitate person-centred communication.

Person-centred communication is particularly important in healthcare practice (Epstein and Street, 2007, p. 17) as this can benefit health outcomes by:
- fostering healing relationships;
- exchanging information;
- responding to emotions;
- managing uncertainty;
- enabling self-management.

Effective and person-centred communication skills are also key to assessment and care planning processes. Older people appreciate healthcare professionals using a structure to the history-taking interview by explaining the reasons for the consultation and what it will involve (Cochran, 2005). The Calgary-Cambridge module of interview structure (Figure 3.1) is one way in which a healthcare professional can undertake a patient's interview in a structured manner. However, for older people, it is also important that they are able to share something about themselves and their life history, alongside the other information gathered, as this will help to establish rapport and facilitate the person-centred approach to communication.

Achieving person-centred communication, however, requires the healthcare professional to be aware of their behaviours and responses, acknowledging that sometimes they will unintentionally affect communication processes. More specifically, healthcare professionals need to be aware of their

Nursing Older People at a Glance, First Edition. Edited by Josie Tetley, Nigel Cox, Kirsten Jack and Gary Witham.
© 2018 John Wiley & Sons, Ltd. Published 2018 by John Wiley & Sons, Ltd.

non-verbal as well as their verbal communication in order to prevent conflicting messages being given to the patient.

Verbal communication is communicating to other people using words or noises to get your message across to the person you are communicating with. **Non-verbal communication** is communicating to people using sign language, hand gestures, body language, such as facial gestures, smiling and eye contact. While both are important, they may need particular consideration and adaptation when working with older people.

Communicating with older people

Sensory changes occur with the normal ageing process. In particular hearing and vision changes can have a direct and significant impact on communication and cognitive processing as follows.

Hearing loss associated with normal ageing begins after the age of 50 due to cells being lost and not replaced within the inner ear. These changes initially lead to the inability to hear high-frequency sounds such as f, s, th, sh and ch. Lower frequency sounds are preserved for longer.

When caring for an older adult it is important to bear in mind the impact that background noise has on a person's ability to communicate and interact with others. This may also impact on the patient's ability to understand important information about their health condition if information is being delivered within a noisy healthcare setting.

Vision normally declines as a person ages – colours become dimmer and images are less distinctive. More seriously, age-related vision problems, such as cataracts, glaucoma and age-related macular degeneration, can cause blindness. Changes in vision have implications for communication, as they may affect the older person's ability to see the healthcare professional smiling, nodding their head or other non-verbal communication.

Communication skills

- Make sure spectacles, hearing aids and dentures are for the right person, and are clean, working and worn.
- Make sure you have the person's attention before speaking.
- Don't shout but speak clearly and reduce background noise.
- Allow the patient time to respond.
- Avoid child-like or patronising language.

Information-giving skills (Edwards, 2010)

- Check what the person already knows.
- Give information in small chunks – pause.
- Use clear and simple terms.

- Avoid detail unless requested.
- Pause to allow information to sink in.
- Wait for a response.
- Check what has been understood.
- Negotiate to continue.
- Check the patient's understanding.

Listening skills (Bach, 2015)

- Pay attention, use your body language to show you are listening.
- Use reflection.
- Allow the speaker to finish what they are saying.
- Acknowledge what has been said and check you have understood correctly.
- Summarise what has been said.
- Use empathy to encourage further disclosure of concerns.

Summary

While effective and person-centred communication can have positive outcomes for both healthcare professionals and patients it is also important to plan ahead and consider any barriers that might impact on the person's ability to communicate such as: lack of privacy, noise and distractions. Effective communication also involves listening to what the person is saying and checking that they have understood any instructions they are being given – whether this is about medication regimens, self-management advice or future appointments. When working with older people the use of verbal and non-verbal communication may need to be adapted to compensate for sensory changes. Strategies that can help develop a rapport with the person are likely to improve the overall quality of interactions with the older person.

References

Bach, S. (2015) *Communication and Interpersonal Skills in Nursing*. Transforming nursing practice series. London: Learning Matters.

Cochran, P. (2005) Acute care for elders prevents functional decline. *Nursing* 35(10): 70–71.

Edwards, M. (2010) *Communication Skills for Nurses: A practical guide on how to achieve successful consultations*. London: Quay Books.

Epstein, R.M. and Street, R.L. (2007) *Patient-Centered Communication in Cancer Care: Promoting Healing and Reducing Suffering*. NIH publication no. 076225. Bethesda, MD: National Cancer Institute.

Kurtz, S.M., Silverman, J.D., Benson, J. and Draper, J. (2003) Marrying content and process in clinical method teaching: enhancing the Calgary-Cambridge guides. *Academic Medicine* 78: 802–809.

4 Compassion

Figure 4.1 The BOND framework. Source: Adapted from Baughan and Smith (2013). Reproduced with permission of Taylor & Francis Group.

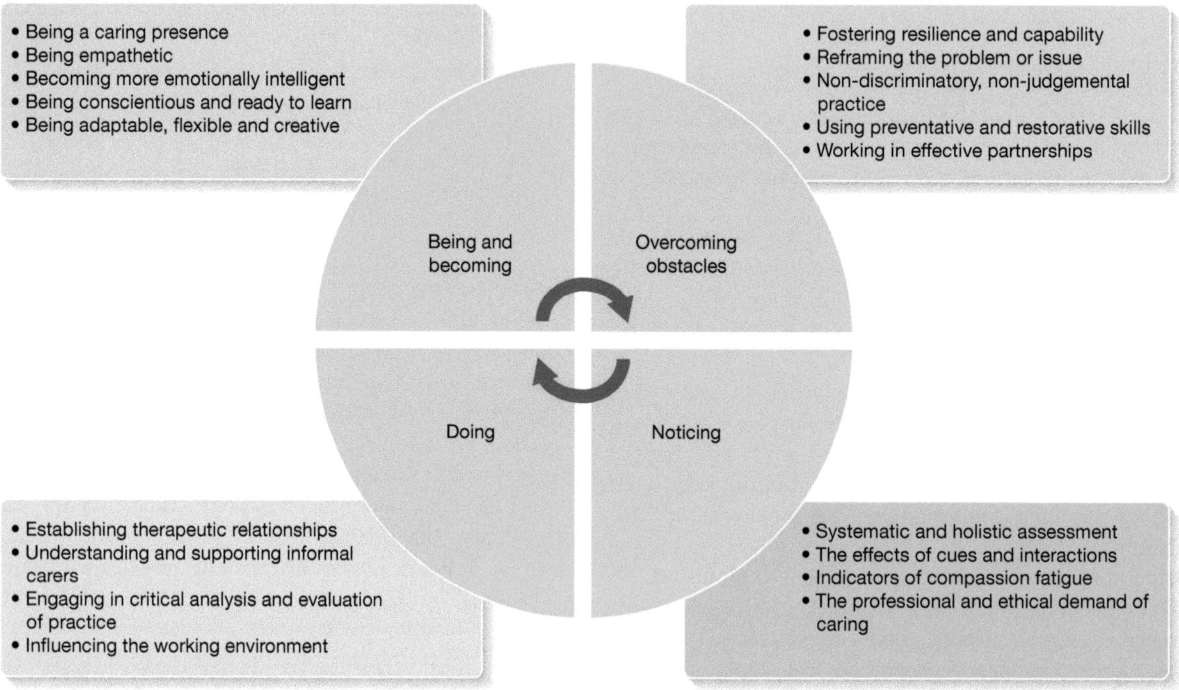
• Being a caring presence
• Being empathetic
• Becoming more emotionally intelligent
• Being conscientious and ready to learn
• Being adaptable, flexible and creative
• Fostering resilience and capability
• Reframing the problem or issue
• Non-discriminatory, non-judgemental practice
• Using preventative and restorative skills
• Working in effective partnerships
Being and becoming
Overcoming obstacles
Doing
Noticing
• Establishing therapeutic relationships
• Understanding and supporting informal carers
• Engaging in critical analysis and evaluation of practice
• Influencing the working environment
• Systematic and holistic assessment
• The effects of cues and interactions
• Indicators of compassion fatigue
• The professional and ethical demand of caring

Table 4.1 The nature of compassion. Source: Adapted from Van der Cingel (2011).

Dimension	
Attentiveness	Consciously showing interest in whatever is important to the other person; supported by appropriate gestures and touch
Listening	Keeping silent and encouraging the patient to tell their story; being willing to hear what is being said
Confronting	Assessing the meaning of the loss to the patient and validating their emotions
Involvement	Recognising and sharing emotions, to form a bond between the patient and the nurse
Helping attitudes	Helping with and anticipating basic needs, suggesting different ways to deal with issues and promoting independence
Presence	Being there and noticing what is happening with the patient. Noticing the need to be there
Understanding	Trying our best to understand patients' feelings and showing this understanding to them

Nursing Older People at a Glance, First Edition. Edited by Josie Tetley, Nigel Cox, Kirsten Jack and Gary Witham.

Compassion is a complex phenomenon and difficult to define. Compassion is considered by some to be subjective in nature (Dewar *et al.*, 2011), although it is a central concept in the Nursing and Midwifery Code (Nursing and Midwifery Council, 2015). Compassion is also one of the values of the 'Six C's' of nursing, the vision for the future launched by the Chief Nursing Officer (CNO) for England (Cummings and Bennett, 2012). Described as 'intelligent kindness' (Cummings and Bennett, 2012, p. 13), it is viewed as central to how people perceive the care provided.

Compassion has been shown to be a particularly valuable phenomenon when caring for older people and one that supports high-quality care in this setting (Van der Cingel, 2011). A more comprehensive definition is suggested by Dewar *et al.* (2011, p. 32), who suggest compassion is:

> *...the way in which we relate to human beings. It can be nurtured and supported. It involves noticing another person's vulnerability, experiencing an emotional reaction to this and acting in some way with them, in a way that is meaningful for people. It is defined by the people who give it and receive it, and therefore interpersonal processes that capture what it means to people are an important element of its promotion.*

For nurses to be able to show compassion to older people, there is a need to engage in an emotional relationship with them (Freshwater and Cahill, 2010). We also need to recognise its individual meaning.

Model of compassionate care

Baughan and Smith (2013) propose an initial framework that can be used to support understanding of the nature of compassionate care provision and enhance skills in this aspect of practice (Figure 4.1). The authors acknowledge that the framework is a basic prompt for thinking and should be used as a basis for further learning development. For example, 'Caring by being and becoming' signifies our ongoing development as practitioners and the fact that we change over time, based on our experiences and knowledge.

What is compassion from an older person's perspective?

It is important to know how older people perceive compassionate care provision. Based on a qualitative research study of older people with a chronic disease, Van der Cingel (2011) proposed a structure based on seven recognisable dimensions, taken from both the patients' and nurses' perspectives (Table 4.1).

Developing compassionate environments

Consideration of frameworks is important to support the development of compassionate practice. Nurses have a responsibility to model compassionate behaviours to patients and other staff members. Understanding what older people want is central to us developing appropriate compassionate practice, and one way this can be supported is through engagement in 'appreciative caring conversations' (Dewar and Nolan, 2013). Talking about care with patients and relatives is important if we are going to fully understand what is important to them. Central to this process is the nurse's ability to remain self-aware, as understanding ourselves is essential if we are going to begin to understand others. Developing self-awareness can be achieved by ongoing reflection on our thoughts and feelings. Bramley and Matiti (2014) suggest that gaining an understanding of the impact of uncompassionate action is a powerful motivator for change on an individual and organisational level. Clinical supervision provides an opportunity for practitioners to reflect on their practice and discuss difficult situations with a view to developing compassionate practice and culture (Care Quality Commission, 2013).

Supporting compassionate care

Experiential learning can be helpful to support development of compassionate practice. Reflecting on events can help us to understand ourselves in different ways. Through this process, new opportunities to promote compassionate practice can be revealed. Feedback from trusted colleagues can support compassionate practice development. Used effectively, constructive feedback can help us to learn more about ourselves and the ways we practise. Using a positive role model can also support our compassionate practice as we can observe the role model's behaviour, and use this to inform our own development.

References

Baughan, J. and Smith, A. (2013) *Compassion, Caring and Communication: Skills for Nursing Practice*, 2nd edn. Abingdon/New York: Routledge.

Bramley, L. and Matiti, M. (2014) How does it really feel to be in my shoes? Patients' experiences of compassion within nursing care and their perceptions of developing compassionate nurses. *Journal of Clinical Nursing* 23: 2790–2799.

Care Quality Commission (2013) *Supporting Information and Guidance: Supporting Effective Clinical Supervision*. London: CQC.

Cummings, J. and Bennett, V. (2012) Compassion in Practice. Department of Health; NHS Commissioning Board. Available at: https://www.england.nhs.uk/wp-content/uploads/2012/12/compassion-in-practice.pdf (accessed 15 September 2017).

Dewar, B. and Nolan, M. (2013) Caring about caring: Developing a model to implement compassionate relationship centred care in an older people care setting. *International Journal of Nursing Studies* 50(9): 1247–1258.

Dewar, B., Pullin, S. and Tocheris, R. (2011) Valuing compassion through definition and measurement. *Nursing Management* 17(9): 32–37.

Freshwater, D. and Cahill, J. (2010) Care and Compromise: developing a conceptual model for work related stress. *Journal of Research in Nursing* 15(2): 173–183.

Nursing and Midwifery Council (2015) The Code. London: Nursing and Midwifery Council.

Van der Cingel, M. (2011) Compassion in care: a qualitative study of older people with a chronic disease and nurses. *Nursing Ethics* 18: 672–685.

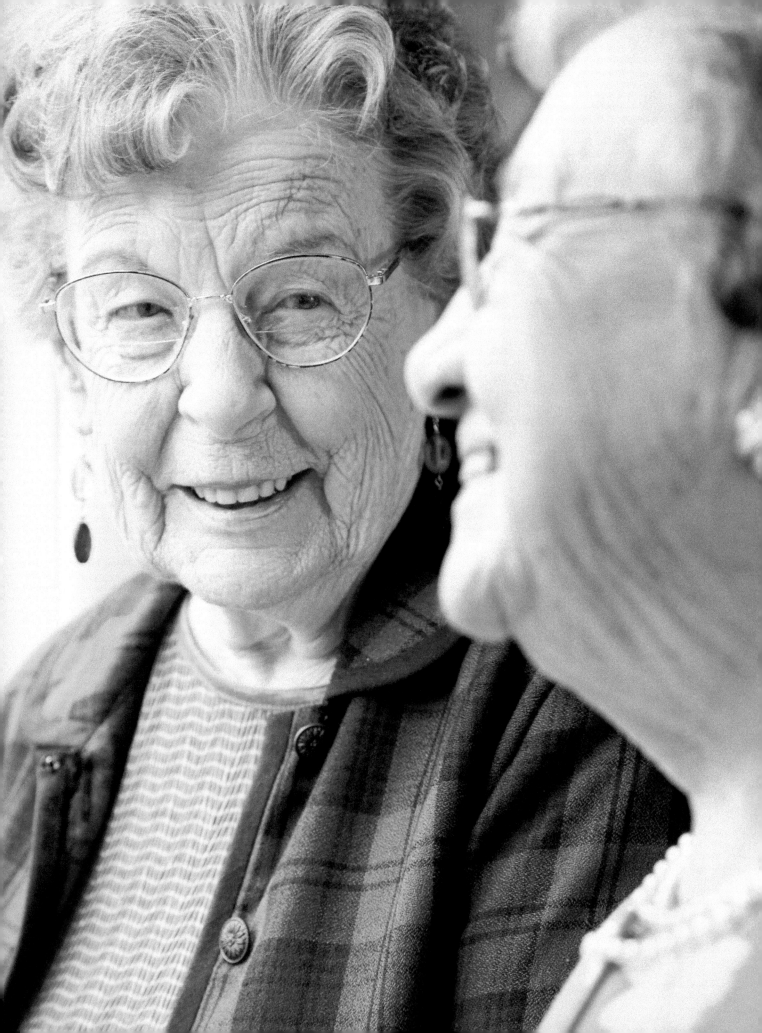

Quality of life in practice

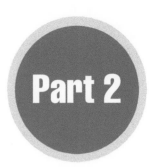

Part 2

Chapters

5 Quality of life

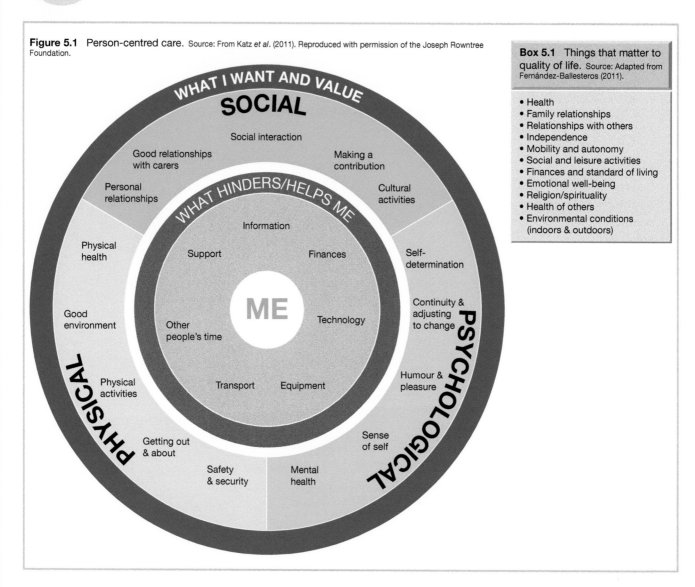

Figure 5.1 Person-centred care. Source: From Katz *et al.* (2011). Reproduced with permission of the Joseph Rowntree Foundation.

Box 5.1 Things that matter to quality of life. Source: Adapted from Fernández-Ballesteros (2011).

- Health
- Family relationships
- Relationships with others
- Independence
- Mobility and autonomy
- Social and leisure activities
- Finances and standard of living
- Emotional well-being
- Religion/spirituality
- Health of others
- Environmental conditions (indoors & outdoors)

What is quality of life (QOL)?

People have always been interested in quality of life (QOL). The ancient Greeks equated QOL with happiness, and today it is recognised that QOL involves psychological, social and environmental factors (Fernández-Ballesteros, 2011). While people will have different views about QOL, both public and professional concepts of quality of life are broadly similar and feature key aspects (Box 5.1).

Quality of life and the individual

While the elements noted in Box 5.1 highlight important aspects of QOL, the *experience* of quality in any, and all, of these is subjective and personal. For some older people, ageing can be a positive experience that provides renewed opportunities for learning,

social interaction, recreation and support for younger family members. However, for others, the experience of ageing might reduce opportunities, either directly (due to their own increasing frailty and dependence on others) or the need to care for a partner or family member who is also ageing. Some older people may also struggle financially, which can further limit choices.

Having choices

Although physical and cognitive capacities may change, as people get older many will still describe themselves as 'feeling 25 years old inside'. Accepting limitations can be important to self-esteem and quality of life but this does not mean that people want to 'give-up' or be sidelined. Doing something meaningful and having freedom of choice is essential. In a residential

Nursing Older People at a Glance, First Edition. Edited by Josie Tetley, Nigel Cox, Kirsten Jack and Gary Witham.
© 2018 John Wiley & Sons, Ltd. Published 2018 by John Wiley & Sons, Ltd.

setting, for example, choices may be offered around things such as clothing, food and the time someone goes to bed; offering choices about treatment options may also be considered, where possible.

Social activities

Loneliness and social isolation can be problematic for older people (Corbi *et al.*, 2015), with nearly half (46%) of those aged 80 or over reportedly feeling lonely (ONS, 2013). Within their capacities, people still want to do the same things they did when they were younger. Various studies (e.g. Hjaltadóttir and Gústafsdóttir, 2007; Hughes and Moore, 2012) identify that older people place value on their relationships with family and friends, physical care and safe environments.

Whether people stay in their own homes or are in residential accommodation (sheltered housing or nursing homes), maintaining everyday activities is vital and people should continue with existing interests as they grow older. Social get-togethers, meeting friends, pursuing hobbies, volunteering, shopping, gardening, going to church, clubs or night classes should be encouraged, and supported if help is needed, for example, with a person's mobility (Hughes and Moore, 2012).

Safety

Another important element that affects QOL for older people is safety. This might be particularly important in residential settings as people are living together in close proximity. Privacy and personal space are important. People may need to be protected from the unpredictable behaviour of other residents, if this arises, and privacy ensured, for example, by preventing people from wandering into private rooms.

Physical health

Another aspect of maintaining QOL is to ensure that older people's physical health is conserved, and that appropriate treatment of pain or other physical symptoms is provided (Hjaltadóttir and Gústafsdóttir, 2007). It should not be assumed that older people should simply 'put up' with poor health. Rehabilitation exercises and general physical activity are important too, as these can help maintain and improve an individual's independence. Where someone has a cognitive impairment (e.g. due to dementia), it is very important to be particularly vigilant about physical care needs: they may forget if they have had something to eat or drink, and may not be able to tell someone if they are in pain. It is therefore important to observe for signs and symptoms such as agitation or restlessness (Achterberg *et al.*, 2013).

Implications for practice – how might we work towards quality of life?

It is particularly important that older people are not seen as a burden. Person-centred and holistic care is important, and kindness, care and compassion are essential when caring for older people. People are likely to become distressed if they feel rushed, so supporting people with their activities of daily living (e.g. washing, dressing, toileting and eating) in an unhurried manner is important. Nurses and carers should focus on what people can do, not what they cannot do (Hughes and Moore, 2012).

Supporting staff to support older people's needs

It is important for staff to act as advocates for older people, helping them to voice their concerns. By having conversations with older people, we can gain an understanding of what they want from their life, not just what they want from services or care. Figure 5.1 shows a framework that can be used to guide conversation. It is important that this is not used simply as a 'checklist'. Instead, it should be used to encourage *person-led* conversation. Of course, people have different needs and desires, and what emerges from the conversation will vary from person to person.

Conclusion

An essential component of maintaining QOL is to place the individual at the centre of any discussions about what happens to them. This is achieved through conversations, negotiations and relationship building to establish ways in which care can be given to suit the individual, not making assumptions about preferences and abilities, nor focusing solely on the physical aspects of their care. The aim should be to maintain existing ways of living, in so far as practicable: this requires carers to be creative and inventive (Hjaltadóttir and Gústafsdóttir, 2007).

Putting a person at the centre of their care involves treating people as individuals: talking to older people, their family and friends, and their carers, about the things *they* enjoy doing. It also entails involving older people in decision-making and, whenever possible, providing people with choices regarding what they do and what will happen to them. Social and psychological needs should also be recognised and addressed alongside physical needs, for instance by helping people carry on with the hobbies and social activities they have enjoyed throughout their life.

References

Achterberg, W.P., Pieper, M.J.C., van Dalen-Kok, A., de Waal, M.W.M., Husebo, B.S., Lautenbacher, S., *et al.* (2013) Pain management in patients with dementia. *Clinical Interventions in Aging* 8: 1471–1482; doi: 10.2147/CIA.S36739.

Corbi, G., Grattagliano, I., Ivshina, E., Ferrara, N., Solimeno-Cipriano, A. and Pietro-Campobasso, C. (2015) Elderly abuse: risk factors and nursing role. *Internal Emergency Medicine* 10: 297–303.

Fernández-Ballesteros, R. (2011) Quality of life in old age: problematic issues. *Applied Research in Quality of Life* 6: 21–40.

Hjaltadóttir, I., and Gústafsdóttir, M. (2007) Quality of life in nursing homes: perception of physically frail elderly residents. *Scandinavian Journal of Caring Sciences* 21: 48–55.

Hughes K. and Moore, S. (2012) Quality of life versus quality of care: elderly people and their experience of care in South Australian residential facilities. *Practice: Social Work in Action* 24(5): 275–285.

Katz, J., Holland, C., Peace, S. and Taylor, E (ed. Blood, I.) (2011) *A Better Life – what older people with high support needs value*. York: Joseph Rowntree Foundation/The Open University.

ONS (2013) *Measuring National Well-being – Older people and loneliness, 2013*. London: Office for National Statistics (ONS). Available at: http://www.ons.gov.uk/ons/rel/wellbeing/measuring-national-well-being/older-people-and-loneliness/art-measuring-national-well-being–older-people-and-loneliness.html (accessed 15 September 2017).

6 Nutrition and hydration

Figure 6.1 The importance of hydration.

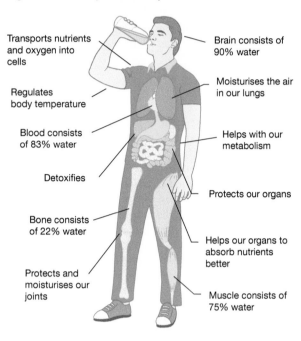

Transports nutrients and oxygen into cells

Regulates body temperature

Blood consists of 83% water

Detoxifies

Bone consists of 22% water

Protects and moisturises our joints

Brain consists of 90% water

Moisturises the air in our lungs

Helps with our metabolism

Protects our organs

Helps our organs to absorb nutrients better

Muscle consists of 75% water

Figure 6.2 Organs of the digestive system.
Source: From Peate and Muralitharan (2015). Reproduced with permission of John Wiley & Sons, Ltd.

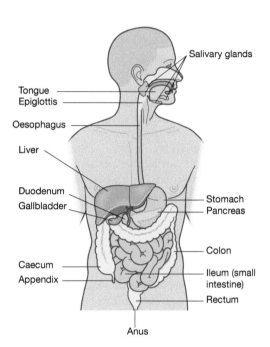

Salivary glands

Tongue
Epiglottis

Oesophagus

Liver

Duodenum
Gallbladder

Caecum
Appendix

Stomach
Pancreas

Colon

Ileum (small intestine)

Rectum

Anus

Table 6.1 Age-related gastrointestinal changes and outcomes for older adults. Source: Adapted from Heath and Sturdy (2009).

Change	Outcome
Decreased taste acuity	Diminished taste and reduced enjoyment of food leading to reduced intake
Decreased saliva production	Xerostomia (dry mouth), soreness, choking
Brittle teeth	Decay and loss of teeth
Receding gums	Difficulty in chewing
Articulation of upper and lower jaw	Difficulty in chewing
Decreased oesophageal peristalsis	Dysphagia, feeling of fullness and heartburn
Decreased gastric secretions	Indigestion – reduced intrinsic factor essential for vitamin B12 absorption, pernicious anaemia

Nursing Older People at a Glance, First Edition. Edited by Josie Tetley, Nigel Cox, Kirsten Jack and Gary Witham.
© 2018 John Wiley & Sons, Ltd. Published 2018 by John Wiley & Sons, Ltd.

Why is nutrition and hydration a concern in older people?

Older people are at risk of malnutrition and dehydration as a result of possible decreased physical health and mental fragility. However, adequate nutrition and fluids are fundamental needs that support life and well-being. Improved health indicators for mental cognition, resistance to and faster recuperation from illness and disease, and higher energy levels are also linked to good nutrition and hydration in older people (British Nutrition Foundation, 2016; Helpguide.org, 2016). In addition good hydration is seen to increase emotional well-being and reduce the use of some medications, and is a factor in preventative healthcare (Carter, 2015). Despite irrefutable evidence linking diet and well-being, the British Nutrition Foundation in 2016 reported on national survey data that illustrated daily intakes of fibre, core vitamins and minerals amongst the elderly were well below the average daily intake of the general population and particularly low amongst individuals living in institutions (British Nutrition Foundation, 2016).

The importance of hydration is shown in Figure 6.1 yet despite the importance of adequate hydration, older people are vulnerable to dehydration due to physiological changes occurring as a result of the ageing process; the situation is complicated by many disease states, and mental and physical frailty that can further increase risk of dehydration. Inadequate fluid intake is a major contributor to preventable dehydration. Poor oral intake of fluids can be related to the inability to feed independently and having poor availability and access to fluids. Even mild dehydration adversely affects mental performance and increases feelings of tiredness. Mental functions affected include memory, attention, concentration and reaction time.

Some of the age-related gastrointestinal changes and outcomes for older adults are highlighted in Table 6.1, which is based on work funded by the Department of Health and published in 2009.

Decreased taste can limit fluid intake if it is not enjoyed; however, adequate hydration is dependent on multiple factors. For example, difficulties with swallowing, mobility and sensory impairment provide obstacles to adequate hydration, as does hospitalisation, which can lead to disorientation and possible confusion. There is evidence also to suggest older people will often limit fluid intake for fear of incontinence or disturbed sleep and where this is identified, it can be swiftly addressed with guidance.

How can effective hydration and nutrition be promoted?

To meet both nutritional and hydration needs it is important that older people are screened appropriately to identify if they are at risk, and if referral to specialised healthcare support services is needed. For many it might be best practice to keep a record of food and fluids taken to inform such an assessment and to determine what interventions are required. Despite the many changes occurring as a result of ageing or disease processes associated with the gastrointestinal tract (Figure 6.2) and possible functional difficulties that might limit access to food and fluids; the aim of any intervention package would be directed towards maintaining as much independence as possible with appropriate health and social care interventions.

Simple interventions are important. For example, maintaining an emphasis on the 'normal' and 'social' aspects of eating and drinking and ensuring that there is easy access to a selection of nutritionally balanced foods and drinks throughout the day. The sense of smell and taste are often compromised in older people therefore interventions aimed to stimulate appetite cannot be overemphasised.

Many simple interventions can make a difference to ensure that older people receive adequate nutrition and hydration. The threat to health for older people is clear from many differing sources. Just considering nutrition, a survey of hospitals, care homes and mental health units reported that a quarter of people aged under 70 were at risk of malnutrition, increasing to a third of those aged 85 years or older (Nursing Standard, 2009). These are prevalent concerns, but often small and informed interventions can make a difference.

The older population remains at risk of undernourishment and dehydration, whether they have existing pathological conditions or nor. Continued assessment, monitoring and access to adequate and good food and drink is not optional but essential for ongoing health and well-being.

References

British Nutrition Foundation (2016) Later life. Available at: https://www.nutrition.org.uk/healthyliving/lifestages/later-life.html (accessed 18 September 2017).

Carter, L. (2015) The importance of maintaining good hydration in older people. Nursing in Practice. Available at: http://www.nursinginpractice.com/article/importance-maintaining-good-hydration-older-people (accessed 18 September 2017).

Heath, H. and Sturdy, D. (2009) Nutrition and Older People. *Nursing Standard*. 23, 40:1-15.

Helpguide.org (2016) Staying healthy as you age: Tips for eating well as you age. Available at: https://www.helpguide.org/articles/alzheimers-dementia-aging/staying-healthy-as-you-age.htm (accessed 3 October 2017).

Nursing Standard (2009) Nutrition and older people. *Nursing Standard* 23(40): 3-3.

Peate, I. and Muralitharan N. (2015) *Anatomy and Physiology for Nurses at a Glance*. Oxford: Wiley Blackwell.

7 Hearing and vision

Figure 7.1   The outer and inner ear. Source: Peate and Muralitharan (2015). Reproduced with permission of John Wiley & Sons, Ltd.

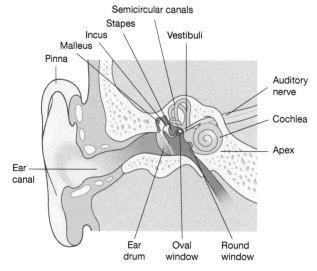

Figure 7.2   Cross-section of the eye. Source: Peate and Muralitharan (2015). Reproduced with permission of John Wiley & Sons, Ltd.

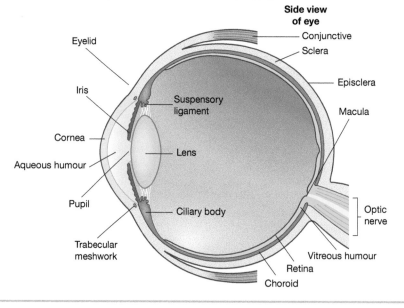

The ear and hearing (Figure 7.1)

Hearing depends on the following phenomena:

- Sound waves enter the outer ear and travel to the eardrum.
- The eardrum vibrates due to the sound and transmits the vibrations to three tiny bones (malleus, incus and stapes).
- The bones vibrate and transmit the vibration to fluid in the cochlea in the inner ear (which is shaped like a snail). In the cochlea is an elastic membrane (basilar membrane) that forms a partition in the cochlea, splitting it into an upper and lower part.
- Once the fluid in the cochlea vibrates a wave travels along the basilar membrane and sensory (hair) cells sitting on top of the membrane are moved by the wave.
- As these hair cells move, tiny hair-like projections bump against overlying structures. They bend, which opens channels in them, allowing chemicals to enter and create an electric signal. Different cells respond to different pitches of sound.
- The auditory nerve carries this signal to the brain, which interprets the signal as sound.

The ear and balance

The vestibular system in the inner ear is sensitive to very small changes in the head's position, detecting circular motion as well as straight line motion, such as stopping or turning, which is important for balance. Along with other areas of the sensory system, the brain keeps track of the position of all elements of our body, as well as our position in space.

Nursing Older People at a Glance, First Edition. Edited by Josie Tetley, Nigel Cox, Kirsten Jack and Gary Witham.
© 2018 John Wiley & Sons, Ltd. Published 2018 by John Wiley & Sons, Ltd.

Age-related changes in hearing

Age related hearing loss (presbyacusis) occurs gradually in most people as they get older. Around a third of people aged between 65 and 74 have some hearing loss. Hearing loss can make it difficult to understand others, to feel part of a conversation, to hear warnings or respond to alerts such as the telephone, and can ultimately make the person feel very isolated.

Many factors contribute to hearing loss such as hypertension and diabetes, as well as changes in the inner ear. Long-term exposure to high levels of noise can damage the hair cells, which do not regenerate. Most elderly people have a combination of age-related hearing loss and **noise-induced hearing loss**.

While most causes of hearing loss cannot be cured, as the sound must first go down a narrow tube, and this tube can block with waxy secretions, the first thing that should be done in hearing loss is to check the patency of this tube. Hearing loss should also be assessed by an audiologist or ear nose and throat physician, so that reversible causes of hearing loss can be identified and if necessary hearing aids prescribed to maximise hearing. There are a number of different types of hearing aids, including those that fit around the ear and those that are barely visible and fit in the ear canal.

Things to consider:
• Some hearing loss is a normal part of ageing. While it cannot be reversed, it can be helped with hearing aids.
• Hearing does not normally deteriorate quickly. Any sudden loss of hearing should be investigated. It may be just a plug of wax in the ear canal, but it may be an indication of more serious disease.
• Hearing aids only work if they fit well and they are worn. It can take a little time for the person to get used to wearing hearing aids. It can be felt to be stigmatising, or the person may feel it is confirmation that they are 'old' so there may be some resistance. Encouragement is often required while getting used to the aids.
• Batteries need replacing regularly; a stock should be kept so that the person is not disadvantaged and isolated by hearing less than they are able to.
• Not being able to hear significantly reduces quality of life.

Balance and falls

Changes in hearing, vision and the vestibular system can resulting in balance problems and falling. Changes in vision are not often considered as a cause of falling and any falls assessment should include vision and balance tests (College of Optometrists/British Geriatrics Society, 2011; NICE, 2013).

The eye and vision (Figure 7.2)

The eye is almost spherical, measuring around 2.4 cm in diameter, and sits in a bony orbit, one each side of the nose. It is a hollow sphere with a number of structures whose role is to focus light onto the back of the eye where it is transformed into electrical signals which go, via the optic nerve, to the brain.

In the eye:
• The cornea forms part of the outermost coat of the eye. It is transparent and its role is to refract (bend) light to a focus on the retina.
• The lens assists in this process and is able to change shape up until about age 50, to allow focusing for near vision as well as distance.
• As the cornea and lens are transparent and without a blood supply, their nutrition comes from aqueous, or aqueous humour, produced by the ciliary body.
• Aqueous is produced continuously and drains continuously through the trabecular meshwork and canal of Schlemm. The quantity of aqueous helps the eye to keep its shape.
• When light reaches the retina, it stimulates photoreceptor cells known as rods and cones (from their shape). The light reacts with a chemical and an electrical signal results, which goes from the photoreceptor, through a network of nerve cells and axons to the optic nerve.
• The optic nerve provides the route to the brain for interpretation of the nerve impulse into what we know as vision.

Ageing and vision

The eyes change as the body ages and some of these changes result in physiological or disease processes causing reduction in vision. Untreatable vision loss is **not** an inevitable consequence of ageing and any vision loss should be investigated.

As the eyes age, many individuals require a change in glasses prescription. Even those who have never worn glasses are likely to need them as they get older. All older people must be encouraged to have an eye test by an optometrist at least every 2 years, or if any change is noticed.

As the lens ages, it gets denser and lets less light through. As it starts to affect vision, this is known as **cataract**.

Insidious (gradual) loss of peripheral and then central vision can be caused by **glaucoma**. This is an imbalance between the production and drainage of aqueous, resulting a higher than normal pressure in the eye and damage to the nerve tissue making up the retina and optic nerve. It is treatable and damage can often be arrested by the use of prescribed eyedrops. It will be detected during a routine eye test by an optometrist.

Loss of central vision should be investigated very promptly as it can be a sign of underlying disease, but also of **age-related macular degeneration**, some forms of which are treatable.

Things to consider:
• Untreatable vision loss is **not** an inevitable consequence of ageing and any vision loss should be investigated.
• Vision does not normally deteriorate quickly so this should be investigated promptly. As it is the brain, rather than the eye that interprets the world for the person, any sudden change in vision or perception might be an indication of brain dysfunction such as stroke.
• A cataract extraction takes around 30 minutes, but needs visual rehabilitation (see http://www.nhs.uk/conditions/Cataract-surgery/Pages/Introduction.aspx).
• Eyedrops are drugs, some of which are extremely powerful and toxic. They should be treated as any other prescribed drug. Missed doses can cause untreatable vision loss.
• Missed outpatient appointments can also result in lost vision; as an advocate for the patient, the carer(s) must make sure outpatient appointments are both made and kept.
• Not being able to see significantly reduces quality of life.

References

College of Optometrists/British Geriatrics Society (2011) The importance of vision in preventing falls. London: College of Optometrists/British Geriatrics Society. Available at: http://www.bgs.org.uk/fallsresources-307/subjectreference/fallsandbones/visionfalls (accessed 18 September 2017).

NHS Choices (2016) Cataract Surgery. Available at: http://www.nhs.uk/conditions/Cataract-surgery/Pages/Introduction.aspx (accessed 18 September 2017).

NICE (2013) Falls in older people: assessing risk and prevention. Clinical Guideline CG161. National Institute for Health and Care Excellence. Available at: https://www.nice.org.uk/Guidance/cg161 (accessed 18 September 2017).

Peate, I. and Muralitharan, N. (2015) *Anatomy and Physiology for Nurses at a Glance*. Oxford: Wiley Blackwell.

8 Pain

Figure 8.1 The assessment cycle.

Look...
- At the person's behaviour
- At their posture or body language
- At how they hold themselves or move – or even IF they move

Listen...
- To what they or their carers are telling you
- To the tone of the patient's voice as they speak
- To what they don't tell, as much as what they do

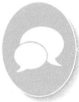

Ask...
- The patient what is wrong
- Them where it hurts and what kind of pain it is
- Carers/friends if this is usual behaviour for them

Believe....
- What the patient tells you about their pain
- That older people are more than their medical diagnosis
- That you can help them

Key points

- Take a clear history, assess pain carefully, and remember there may be several different pain types.
- Not all patients can use a simple pain scale; observe facial expressions, mobility and involve family and carers where possible.
- Think about words such as 'sore', 'hurt' and 'comfort' and what they might mean.
- Don't consider pain in isolation from other comorbidities.
- There are a wide range of medications available.
- Don't be afraid to use non-pharmacological treatments such as heat, cold, positioning, and so forth.
- Ask for help when you are not sure what to do.
- Give the medication, and make sure you return to check if it has had the desired effect – from the patient's point of view, not your own.

Nursing Older People at a Glance, First Edition. Edited by Josie Tetley, Nigel Cox, Kirsten Jack and Gary Witham.
© 2018 John Wiley & Sons, Ltd. Published 2018 by John Wiley & Sons, Ltd.

The purpose of this chapter is to introduce some of the issues that need to be considered when caring for an older person in pain. Pain is described as an 'unpleasant sensory or emotional experience associated with actual or potential tissue damage or described in terms of such damage' (Merskey and Bogduk, 1994). An individual's perception of pain is influenced by a number of factors including their expectations, culture, mood, social support, setting, fear of side effects, and past medical history. Nonetheless, it is important from the outset to emphasise one fundamental point, namely:

If an experience, intervention or biological disorder is painful at the age of 5, 15 or 30, it will be equally painful at 65, 70 or 90. Age is never a reason for not treating reported pain.

Having made that point it can be acknowledged that there are specific preconceptions that can hamper the effective pain management of this particular client group, and the more common of these are briefly deliberated on below.

• *Pain is an inevitable part of growing old.*

There are research studies that suggest that older people themselves expect their pain level to increase as they get older (e.g. Sarkisian *et al.*, 2002), and certainly musculoskeletal changes can contribute to significant chronic pain in this age group. From a nursing perspective, it is important to collect a comprehensive pain history in order to understand levels of 'everyday pain' and how these may compare with any new pain that requires treatment and also how such treatment may impact on or be impacted by existing medication. For example, if a patient is on a high dose of opioids for cancer, discontinuing such treatment in order to give smaller levels of opioid for postoperative pain is inappropriate and inefficient.

• *Older people interpret pain differently and are often stoic about their pain.*

A number of older people will use the experiences of their contemporaries as a yardstick by which to measure their own pain. Schofield (2007) notes that older people in her study would dwell less on their own pain and more on being thankful that they were fitter than some of their contemporaries. In addition, some older people come from a generation where discussing feelings was not socially acceptable, which may render them reluctant to disclose pain even in a healthcare setting. From a nursing perspective this means that self reports of 'I'm fine' may need further skilled probing to elicit a more realistic pain assessment (Figure 8.1).

• *Older people need less analgesia.*

How the body metabolises medication does indeed change over time and there is concern expressed by some authors about the long-term effects on organ systems of continued analgesic use in older people (Davison, 2015), especially around the use of non-steroidal anti-inflammatory drugs, known as NSAIDs (Arneric *et al.*, 2014). There are numerous policies and guidelines, education programmes, new technologies and effective drugs available to guide pain treatment and to ensure that suitable and safe analgesia can be prescribed and administered. Specialists such as pain nurses, anaesthetists, physiotherapists and pharmacists can also help. Skilled nursing observation supported (when possible) by patient reports will allow for the titration of analgesia to effective and safe levels

• *Older people have other morbidities that explain pain behaviour.* Without doubt, older people will present with a number of comorbidities, which may compromise effective pain assessment. There is often a tendency amongst healthcare professionals to assume that the primary diagnosis, for example dementia, is the explanation for aggressive behaviour or in some cases intense screaming. In this instance the best things a nurse can do are (1) listen to the patient's main carer – they will know intimately whether this behaviour is a 'normal' part of the disease process or due to pain; and (2) administer whatever pain relief has been prescribed IMMEDIATELY and follow this up with an assessment 15 minutes later (Finka *et al.*, 2015).

In conclusion, it is clear from the examples we have presented above that the key to effectively managing pain in older people is grounded in comprehensive assessment of pain and pain behaviours coupled with follow-up assessment of effectiveness of any analgesic interventions provided. See Box 8.1.

References

Arneric, S.P., Laird, J.M., Chappell, A.S. and Kennedy, J.D. (2014) Tailoring chronic pain treatments for the elderly: are we prepared for the challenge? *Drug Discovery Today* 19: 8–17.

Davison, S.N. (2015) Pain, analgesics, and safety in patients with CKD. *Clinical Journal of the American Society of Nephrology* 10: 350–352.

Finka, R.M., Gates, R.A. and Montgomery, R.K. (2015) *Pain Assessment*. Oxford: Oxford University Press.

Merskey, H. and Bogduk, N. (1994) *Taxonomy of Pain Terms & Definitions*. Seattle: IASP Press.

Sarkisian, C.A., Hays, R.D. and Mangione, C.M. (2002) Do older adults expect to age successfully? The association between expectations regarding aging and beliefs regarding healthcare seeking among older adults. *Journal of the American Geriatrics Society* 50: 1837–1843.

Schofield, P. (ed.) (2007) The Management of Pain in Older People. John Wiley & Sons, Ltd.

9 Sleep

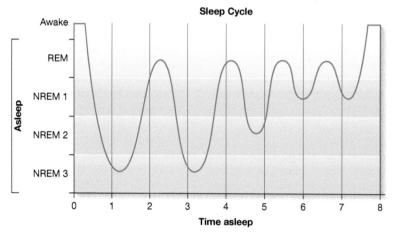

Figure 9.1 The sleep cycle. Source: Reproduced with permission of the Sleep Council.

Table 9.1 Factors affecting sleep in a hospital setting.

Internal Factors	External Factors
• Worry over current condition • Pain (sleep deprivation and pain, acute or chronic, have an adverse effect on each other) • Fear over potential diagnosis • Concern over impending treatments such as theatre or other invasive or non-invasive interventions	• Noise (staff and patients) • Observations (unwell patients require more frequent observations, which in turn can cause a reduction in sleep) • Light (acutely ill patients are more frequently exposed to bright light) • Smells • Other patients (wandering or intervention by nurses)

Nursing Older People at a Glance, First Edition. Edited by Josie Tetley, Nigel Cox, Kirsten Jack and Gary Witham.
© 2018 John Wiley & Sons, Ltd. Published 2018 by John Wiley & Sons, Ltd.

Sleep is a vitally important aspect in all our lives and is required for our health and well-being. If we don't get enough restorative sleep then we can become agitated, confused and unable to concentrate on even the simplest of activities. Sleep is not merely the absence of wakefulness but something much more significant that is complex, multi-dimensional and active (Morin and Espie, 2012). It involves various parts of the brain and numerous hormones either increasing or decreasing in activity and production. Sleep serves an essential function at a cellular level and is influenced by both circadian rhythm and homeostatic processes leading to a propensity to sleep at certain times throughout the day. The circadian rhythm is controlled by cells in the hypothalamus and acts as the body's natural clock, which controls the sleep-wake cycle, body temperature and hormonal levels. However, as we age these rhythms can change leading to alterations in our sleep pattern including reduction of duration of sleep and increased wakefulness throughout the night, thus causing a decrease in restorative sleep. Illness and lifestyle can also lead to changes in sleep patterns – from increased sleepiness when acutely unwell, as the body tries to repair itself, or increased wakefulness during periods of stress and anxiety or if the individual takes stimulants such as caffeine and nicotine prior to going to sleep.

Sleep has been studied for many years and a consistent viewpoint regarding the stages and cycles of sleep is confirmed, although further work continues. These stages are derived from readings produced by the brain during sleep studies detected by EEG (electroencephalography). We move through these stages of sleep through the night in 90-minute cycles each of which includes rapid (REM) and non-rapid eye movement (NREM) stages, with the REM stage increasing as we stay asleep (Figure 9.1).

How much is enough sleep?

Reading (2013) suggests that around 90% of adults require at least 7 hours of sleep per night, less than this can result in reduced levels of observable alertness even if the subject doesn't feel overly tired. As we age our desire to sleep naturally occurs earlier in the evening at around 30 minutes each decade leading to earlier rising (Reading, 2013). Lack of effective sleep, less than 6 or 7 hours per night, has been objectively proven to increase susceptibility to the common cold (rhinovirus) in a wide range of adults (18–55) (Prather et al., 2015). Although this study excluded an older age group it can be surmised that given as we age our sleep pattern shortens and effective sleep duration is reduced, the older person can become more susceptible to illness especially the common cold. It was also found that older, sleep-deprived patients have an increased mortality, although when looking at these results the increased morbidity of older populations must be taken into account (Silva et al., 2016).

Sleep latency (time taken to fall asleep), sleep duration and the number of cycles that an individual experiences are commonly termed sleep 'architecture', and it is a disruption in this that can cause both short- and long-term effects. Sleep in a hospital setting can be very difficult to attain and maintain, and hospitalisation can lead to sleep disruption and deprivation (Lee et al., 2007). This can be due to a number of external, or environmental, and internal factors (Table 9.1).

Nurses have a responsibility and ideal opportunity to improve patients' sleep architecture in some very simple and often financially negligible ways:
- Comfort is important; therefore ensuring a relaxing environment can dramatically influence a patient's sleep. Objective measures that can be influenced include heat, noise and light, all of which have been shown to affect a person's ability to attain and maintain sleep.
- If a patient can't fall asleep or wakes, advising them to settle down and go back to sleep may not be the best option. Getting out of bed for a short time and undertaking something relaxing like listening to quiet music or reading may lead to the patient feeling tired enough to fall asleep.
- Encouraging light exercise can also lead to improved sleep architecture along with the myriad of other benefits that this has, although physical activity in the older person in hospital can be severely limited.

Daytime sleepiness is common in the older person and this can be both social and physical in nature, with a propensity to 'cat nap' through the day due to lack of stimulation or medication side effects. This can lead to a realignment of the circadian rhythm causing night-time wakefulness.

Promoting quality sleep in the older person in hospital can be regarded as important as the administration of medication or the dressing of a wound and should be commonplace as part of the holistic role of the nurse.

References

Lee, C.Y., Low, L.P.L. and Twinn, S. (2007) Older men's experience of sleep in the hospital. *Journal of Clinical Nursing* 16: 336–343.

Morin, C.M. and Espie, C.A. (eds) (2012) *The Oxford Handbook for Sleep and Sleep Disorders*. Oxford: Oxford University Press.

Prather, A.A. Janicki-Deverts, D., Hall, M.H. and Cohen, S. (2015) Behaviorally assessed sleep and susceptibility to the common cold. *Sleep* 38: 1353–1359.

Reading, P. (2013) *ABC of Sleep medicine*. Chichester: John Wiley & Sons, Ltd.

Silva, A.A., Mello, R.B., Schaan, C.W., Flavio, D.F., Redline, S. and Fuchs, S.C. (2016) Sleep duration and mortality in the elderly: a systematic review with meta-analysis. *BMJ Open*. Available at: http://bmjopen.bmj.com/content/6/2/e008119.full.pdf+html?sid=84d40d36-141c-45ee-87e7-0f520846aeb1 (accessed 18 September 2017).

Sleep Council. *The Good Night Guide*. Available from http://www.sleepcouncil.org.uk/wp-content/uploads/2013/01/The-Good-Night-Guide.pdf (accessed 18 September 2017).

10 Continence

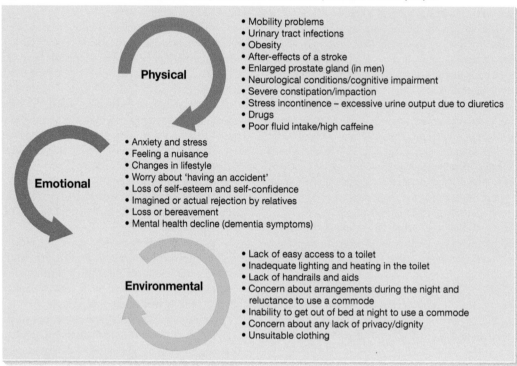

Figure 10.1 Factors that contribute to urinary and faecal continence problems in older people.

Physical
- Mobility problems
- Urinary tract infections
- Obesity
- After-effects of a stroke
- Enlarged prostate gland (in men)
- Neurological conditions/cognitive impairment
- Severe constipation/impaction
- Stress incontinence – excessive urine output due to diuretics
- Drugs
- Poor fluid intake/high caffeine

Emotional
- Anxiety and stress
- Feeling a nuisance
- Changes in lifestyle
- Worry about 'having an accident'
- Loss of self-esteem and self-confidence
- Imagined or actual rejection by relatives
- Loss or bereavement
- Mental health decline (dementia symptoms)

Environmental
- Lack of easy access to a toilet
- Inadequate lighting and heating in the toilet
- Lack of handrails and aids
- Concern about arrangements during the night and reluctance to use a commode
- Inability to get out of bed at night to use a commode
- Concern about any lack of privacy/dignity
- Unsuitable clothing

Table 10.1 NICE (National Institute for Health and Care Excellence) guidelines and quality standards.

Guideline CG49	2007, reviewed 2014	Faecal incontinence in adults: management
Quality Standard QS45	2013	Lower urinary tract symptoms in men
Quality Standard QS77	2015	Urinary continence in women
Guideline NG22	2015	Older people with social care needs and multiple long-term conditions
Readers should explore the full range of guidelines, pathways and standards at: www.nice.org.uk/		

Figure 10.2 Contributing factors for faecal continence problems.

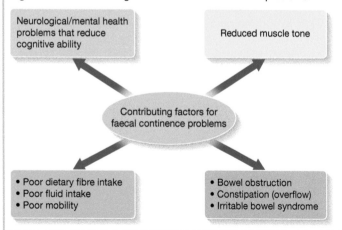

Neurological/mental health problems that reduce cognitive ability

Reduced muscle tone

Contributing factors for faecal continence problems

- Poor dietary fibre intake
- Poor fluid intake
- Poor mobility

- Bowel obstruction
- Constipation (overflow)
- Irritable bowel syndrome

Box 10.1 Continence myths.

- Incontinence is part of the normal ageing process.
- Little can be done for incontinence.
- Toileting residents every 2 hours prevents incontinence.
- Restricting fluids reduces continence problems.

Nursing Older People at a Glance, First Edition. Edited by Josie Tetley, Nigel Cox, Kirsten Jack and Gary Witham.
© 2018 John Wiley & Sons, Ltd. Published 2018 by John Wiley & Sons, Ltd.

Continence problems

Probably one of the biggest setbacks to our self-image and self-confidence would be a continence problem. Whatever our age, it is likely to disrupt our daily routine, self-image and quality of life. The ability to control our bowel and bladder function may range from voiding/staining when coughing or sneezing to no control over urinary or faecal evacuation. Evidence suggests that incontinence may affect between 31% and 70% of older people who live in care homes (Roe *et al.*, 2015), therefore the promotion and maintenance of continence is a priority for all nursing and care staff caring for older people. Prevention, if possible, should be the first consideration. Once identified, a continence problem should not be considered a permanent, enduring situation. Instead, a holistic medical and nursing assessment is the starting point: nursing and care staff need to consider how and why a continence problem has arisen for the older person, and steps taken to limit its escalation (Table 10.1).

The factors contributing to the continence problem need to be identified and assessed thoroughly (Figure 10.1). The multidisciplinary team needs to be fully involved in order for holistic care interventions to be planned, implemented and evaluated (Orrell *et al.*, 2013).

Faecal continence problems pose a significant challenge for both patient and nursing and care staff as the maintenance of continence is an important aspect of an individual's self-image. Roe *et al.* (2015) reported in a systematic review of people in care homes that there was a reluctance of people to report bowel function and control problems to healthcare professionals in the community due to the 'taboo' nature of the subject. This is apparent by the general lack of media exposure to this very sensitive subject (Box 10.1). Qualitative research has demonstrated that health education and promotion for carer staff and family carers, on the topic of faecal continence, can have an impact on maintaining optimal bowel function and continence (Orrell *et al.*, 2013). The contributing factors should be part of the assessment (Figure 10.2). Urinary and faecal continence problems can be symptomatic in advanced dementia, and maintaining a patient's dignity and person-centred care should be paramount (Andrews, 2013; NMC, 2015). Nurses and care staff at all levels need to consider how continence is managed in those who are immobile; absorbent products can be used for long-term management (Nazarko, 2015), and are preferable to catheters, which can cause not only infection but also long-term progressive damage to the urinary tract. In addition to meeting patients' hygiene needs, consideration and compassion are also essential because the emotional impact of incontinence upon the individual may be high. A combination of strategies is more likely to improve continence rather than one single intevention.

Continence care checklist – options and actions

- Holistic medical and nursing assessment.
- Specialist continence services should be considered as early as possible.
- Surgical assessment.
- Pelvic floor exercises.
- Consider prompted voiding programmes.
- Drug therapy.
- Fluid intake/output records are essential.
- Urinary catheters/intermittent, external sheaths (men).
- Incontinence products/devices.
- Personal care a priority.
- Ensure that constipation and faecal impaction are addressed.
- Review medication to identify those that may have an impact on the incontinence.
- Regular evaluation and review.
- Record and review diet.
- Patient-centred care/emotional support.

Products for discreet management of continence problems are becoming readily available, with continence products for both men and women being advertised in popular media. This is hopefully leading to more open acknowledgement of the issues faced by both the sufferer and the care team alike. Promotion and improvement of the level of continence should be the aim: a cure may not be always possible, but supporting and promoting good management remains an integral part of care.

References

Andrews, J. (2013) Maintaining continence in people with dementia. *Nursing Times* 109(27): 20–21.

Nazarko, L. (2015) Use of continence pads to manage urinary continence in older people. *British Journal of Community Nursing* 20(8): 378, 380, 382–384.

NMC (2015) *The Code: Professional Standards of Practice and Behaviour for Nurses and Midwives.* London: Nursing and Midwifery Council.

Orrell, A., McKee, K., Dahlberg, L., Gilhooly, M. and Parker, S. (2013) Improving continence services for older people from the service-providers' perspective: a qualitative interview study. *BMJ Open* 3(7). Available at: http://bmjopen.bmj.com/content/3/7/e002926 (accessed 18 September 2017).

Roe, B., Flanagan, L. and Maden, M. (2015) Systematic review of systematic reviews for the management of urinary incontinence and promotion of continence using conservative behavioural approaches in older people in care homes. *Journal of Advanced Nursing* 71: 1464–1483.

11 End of life care

Figure 11.1 End of life priorities. Source: http://www.ncpc.org.uk/ChoiceOffersConsultation (accessed February 2017). Reproduced with permission of The National Council for Palliative Care (NCPC).

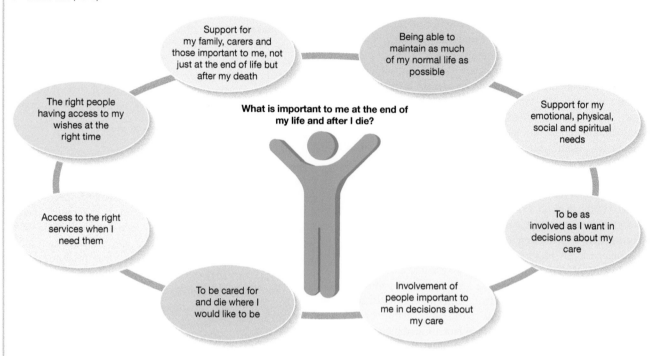

Figure 11.2 A social capital framework. Source: Lewis *et al.* (2013). Reproduced with permission of Elsevier.

Micro/Bonded	Meso/Bridged		Macro/Linked	
(a) Advocate in existing close networks and relations	**(b) Bring about intra-community formal and informal networks and relations**	**(c) Connect with inter-community networks**	**(d) Drive linkages with government institutions and organisations**	
1. Identify and understand the quality and quantity of patient/carer networks and relations. 2. Identify and mobilise family caregiver networks for support for main carer. 3. Identify population subgroups at risk for limited/negative social capital outcomes, e.g. low socioeconomic and cultural groups, female carers.	1. Referral to palliative and general healthcare service agencies, for homecare services. 2. Identify and support possible carer networks beyond immediate family. 3. Primary care providers through 'social prescribing' identify and enable linkages with intra-community network, e.g. neighborhood groups, respite services and volunteer visitor groups.	1. Engage and create partnerships with intersectoral service agencies through (volunteer) community network facilitators, e.g. schools, media groups and government support agencies. 2. Broker support/engagement from community groups and programs, e.g. arts, cultural and religious groups, and internet/web based groups and programs.	1. Peak palliative care providers create partnerships for the development of public infrastructure and social programs and policy. 2. Collaboration between peak palliative care providers and government(s) to communicate policies, programs and legislations which support palliative care populations. 3. Broker reliable resources from government organisations for intra- and inter-community services.	Structural
4. Identify values and levels of trust, reciprocity and motivation for social enagagement.	4. Identify and understand levels of trust and norms for intra-community networks and relations through primary care providers.	3. Identify and understand levels of trust and norms for inter-community networks and through connections with community organisation.	4. Creation of levels of trust and participation which support social cohesion and social inclusion.	Cognitive

Nursing Older People at a Glance, First Edition. Edited by Josie Tetley, Nigel Cox, Kirsten Jack and Gary Witham.
© 2018 John Wiley & Sons, Ltd. Published 2018 by John Wiley & Sons, Ltd.

Box 11.1 Enhancing communication skills.

- Attending communication training courses and workshops has been shown to improve how significant news at the end of life is delivered and dealt with.
- Using tools designed to facilitate conversations about end of life care such as The Conversation Game™ (http://conversationsforlife.co.uk/conversation-game/) or Go Wish (http://www.gowish.org/) card games can be an effective intervention.
- Issues related to advanced care planning should be considered over a number of meetings with a trained professional including adequate time to explore the issues. This should be oriented to the goals of care rather than specific treatment(s).

The End of Life Care Strategy (Department of Health, 2008) provides the framework to enhance end of life care for patients. Education and training, however, are required particularly on prognosis and goals of care with patients and their families at the end of life. Incorporating palliative care earlier in the disease trajectory and implementing a phased transition is an effective approach to support patient care (Gardiner *et al.*, 2011). The publishing of the Neuberger review (2013) of the Liverpool Care Pathway and the subsequent recommendation of the latter's withdrawal has highlighted the complexities of end of life care in recognising dying, maintaining effective communication with both patients and relatives, and issues related to hydration and nutrition at the end of life – all issues important for older people at the end of life. The Leadership Alliance for the Care of Dying People (2014) subsequently set priorities focused on issues related to recognising and communicating dying, and sensitive communication between staff, the dying person and those identified as important to them. It also focused on involvement in decision-making, capacity, the needs of family and others, and planning care.

Communication

The frail elderly can be seen to be in a transitional position between living and dying, with health professionals unsure how to deal with a 'frailing body' in late old age (Nicholson *et al.*, 2012, p. 1430). Effective communication can improve patient understanding, allow access to appropriate services and improve quality of life (Box 11.1). At the end of life, spending time with the person, demonstrating caring, acknowledging fear and reframing hope and honesty in the provision of information is of central importance (Stajduhar *et al.*, 2010). Enabling patients to ask questions that address their concerns may also lead to improvements in communication and subsequent understanding. For health professionals 'being present' rather than 'doing' tasks is a key component of effective communication and needs more validation within practice. Within formalised healthcare there is often a prioritising of service processes rather than a person-centred approach when transitioning between settings at the end of life. Discharge planning can often be initiated without adequate preparation time with insufficient support and information provision regarding available resources. Communicating the purpose of institutional moves for older people is an important issue to address in order to minimise distress.

Health promotion at end of life care

Figure 11.1 highlights the priorities people have towards the end of life; promoting health within the context of a life-limiting condition is an important feature of care. People with life-limiting conditions may experience many different issues including depression, anxiety, social stigma, job loss and family breakdown. Health professionals need to proactively support older people in order to address these potential issues and maintain quality of life. This may need to involve the wider community rather than just service provision by expert professions. Nurses need to promote 'death education' in working to normalise death and to resource communities to better prepare for it, rather than focus on routine (often symptom-based) education offered to carers supporting someone at the end of life.

Maintaining social relations and networks is an important element in supporting quality of life at the end of life. Figure 11.2 describes a social capital framework for understanding social contexts in end of life care. It moves from the micro level (A), a person's relationships and social networks, through to (D), the macro level with linkage with national drivers and policymaking bodies. It is important to explore and expand the focus from formalised healthcare delivery to broader resources enabling communities to manage care at the end of life. Sustaining caring relationships is particularly pertinent to older people and requires acknowledgement of those networks in order to facilitate effective partnerships. In establishing this, advocating in existing close networks and relations is a foundational requirement for health professionals to engage in.

References

Department of Health (2008) End of Life Care Strategy. London: Department of Health. Available at: http://www.cpa.org.uk/cpa/End_of_Life_Care_Strategy.pdf (accessed 3 October 2017).

Gardiner, C., Ingleton, C., Gott, M. and Ryan, T. (2011) Exploring the transition from curative care to palliative care: a systematic review of the literature. *BMJ: Supportive Palliative Care* 1: 56–63.

Leadership Alliance for the Care of Dying People (2014) One chance to get it right: improving peoples' experience of care in the last few days and hours of life. London: Department of Health.

Lewis, J.M., DiGiacomo, M., Luckett, T., Davidson, P.M. and Currow, D.C. (2013) A Social Capital Framework for Palliative Care: Supporting health and well-being for people with life-limiting illness and their carers through social relations and networks. *Journal of Pain and Symptom Management* 45: 92–103.

Neuberger, J. (2013) Review of Liverpool Care Pathway for dying patients: More care, Less pathway. London: Department of Health.

Nicholson, C., Meyer, J., Flatley, M., Holman, C. and Lowton, K. (2012) Living on the margin: understanding the experience of living and dying with frailty in old age. *Social Science & Medicine* 75: 1426–1432.

Stajduhar, K.I., Thorne, S.E., McGuinness, L. and Kim-Sing, C. (2010) Patient perceptions of helpful communication in the context of advanced cancer. *Journal of Clinical Nursing* 19: 2039–2047.

12 Sexual health and well-being

Box 12.1 Factors affecting nurses' discussions of sexual health and well-being with older people.

- Lack of confidence to broach the subject.
- Lack of time.
- Interruptions.
- Limited communication skills.
- Negative attitudes.
- Does not identify sexual health as a priority.
- Assumptions that older people are asexual and therefore not at risk of STIs.

Box 12.2 Sexual health difficulties in older people.

- Erectile dysfunction and associated belief that condoms worsen the problem.
- Vaginal dryness/dyspareunia/anorgasmia following menopause.
- Prostate enlargement.
- Comorbidities, including bladder weakness and chronic pain, which may limit physical sexual activity.
- Psychological concerns (including initiating sex and reluctance in conforming to partner's wishes).
- Alcohol-related sexual health difficulties.

Box 12.3 The PLISSIT model. Source: Annon (1976). Reproduced with permission of Taylor & Francis.

Level I – Permission
The environment, organisational cultures, care practices and staff attitudes communicate that sexuality, intimate relationships and sex are integral to life: in other words, 'permission' for these issues to be acknowledged is implicit.

Level II – Limited information
General information is readily available to patients. Nurses are able to offer general information and to refer to specialist advice or services when appropriate.

Level III – Specific suggestions
Nurses offer opportunities to explore issues or problems within a therapeutic relationship. Information, advice or specialist help to address specific issues or problems is available to patients and significant others as appropriate.

Level IV – Intensive therapy
Professionals with specialist qualifications and usually working within specialist teams (such as psychosexual counsellors or specialists in erectile dysfunction) offer intensive therapy over time. Nurses make referrals, support patients and monitor health and well-being on an ongoing basis.

Nursing Older People at a Glance, First Edition. Edited by Josie Tetley, Nigel Cox, Kirsten Jack and Gary Witham.
© 2018 John Wiley & Sons, Ltd. Published 2018 by John Wiley & Sons, Ltd.

Identifying the older person's sexual health needs

Sex is a basic human need. Our sexual health needs are closely linked to our personal identity, and sexual relationships can provide people of all ages with a number of physical, mental and emotional health benefits. Everyone should be able to access sexual health and well-being support where needed; however, services for older people remain fragmented and focus largely on sexual dysfunction and comorbidities, rather than sexual health and well-being.

In the past, discussions around sexual health have been limited, yet despite the shift to more liberal attitudes in recent decades the sexual health needs of older people remain largely unmet. Indeed, it is suggested that some nurses are reluctant to broach the subject of sexual health and well-being with the older age group for reasons that are outlined in Box 12.1. However, these reflect a lack of awareness and do little to challenge age stereotypes with regard to an older person's sexual health and well-being.

The sexual behaviour of older individuals (age 45–74) was included for the first time in the third National Sexual Health and Attitudes Survey (NATSAL-3) (Mercer *et al.*, 2013). Although the range and frequency of sex reduced with age, many older people reported continuing sexual activity in their later years, with 42% of women and 60% of men, aged 65–74 years, identifying at least one sexual partner during the previous year. The results of the survey also suggest that a number of men and women aged over 45 years are engaging in unsafe sexual practices, including multiple partners and inconsistent condom use. Understanding people's sexual behaviours is important as an increasing number of older people find they are single for the first time in many years, due to relationship breakdown or the death of a long-term partner; a lack of awareness of sexual health protection and reluctance to engage in long-term relationships may subsequently result in increased casual sexual encounters. Whilst many older people do not have to consider the need to prevent pregnancy, age does not provide protection from STIs and the 50+ age group now accounts for the fastest growing group of people diagnosed with HIV (Terrence Higgins Trust, 2015).

Sexual health dysfunction and comorbidity

As people age, the risk of comorbidities, which may limit physical sexual activity, increases. A recent report from the English Longitudinal Study of Ageing (Lee *et al.*, 2015) identified a number of reported sexual health difficulties among older people (Box 12.2). Having an understanding of the impact of comorbidities on sexual well-being, health and functioning can enable nurses to develop empathy and support therapeutic relationships with service users. Individuals and couples may be encouraged to consider and explore other aspects of sexuality to meet their need for intimacy, including touch.

Promoting sexual health in older people: the role of the nurse

It is important that nurses take the needs of older people into account when developing and delivering sexual health promotion information. To be an effective sexual health promoter for older persons, nurses must first examine their own attitudes and values around sex and sexuality among older people, to identify and address any assumptions or prejudice. Nurses must also recognise the diversity of sexual orientation represented in the age group.

Nurses must be aware of the potential for discomfort among older persons where discussions around sex and sexuality may be raised. Such discussions require skill and sensitivity, and the following guidance from the Royal College of Nursing (RCN) supports nurses to broach these topics with older people:

> *Nurses should aim to create an atmosphere conducive to uninterrupted discussion, initiating the conversation, using open-ended questions, being non-judgmental, avoiding abbreviations or jargon and being receptive to clues, however subtle, that the person may offer in terms of what is really important to him or her*
>
> RCN (2011, p. 8)

The most important issue appears to be that of 'permission giving' to invite discussions with older people. The use of the Extended-PLISSIT model may support nurses in addressing sexuality and sexual health when working with older people. Developed from the PLISSIT Model (Box 12.3) a key element of the extended model is that permission giving is a core feature, which Taylor and Davis (2006) suggest should precede *each* of the stages of intervention. Giving permission for patients to express their feelings is likely to provoke mixed responses from patients and it is therefore essential that nurses are respectful of the person's response. However, for many patients being given 'permission' to discuss sensitive issues creates an environment where an individual expresses a willingness to discuss the subject, and enables the nurse to identify areas of need and provide age equal sexual health promotion messages.

References

Annon, J. (1976) The PLISSIT model: a proposed conceptual scheme for the behavioural treatment of sexual problems. *Journal of Sex Education Therapy* 2: 1–15.

Lee, D., Nazroo, J., O'Connor, D., Blake, M. and Pendleton, N. (2015) Sexual health and well-being among older men and women in England: findings from the English Longitudinal Study of Ageing. ELSA. Available at: http://www.elsa-project.ac.uk/publicationDetails/id/7548 (accessed 19 September 2017).

Mercer, C.H., Tanton, C., Prah, P. *et al.* (2013) Changes in sexual attitudes and lifestyles in Britain through the life course and over time: findings from the National Surveys of Sexual Attitudes and Lifestyles (Natsal). *Lancet* 382: 1781–1794; doi:10.1016/S0140-6736 (13) 62035-8.

RCN (2011) Older people in care homes: sex, sexuality and intimate relationships. An RCN discussion and guidance document for the nursing workforce. London: Royal College of Nursing.

Taylor, B. and Davis, S. (2006) Using the Extended PLISSIT model to address sexual healthcare needs. *Nursing Standard* 21(11): 35–40.

Terrence Higgins Trust (2015) 50 plus and living with HIV? Available at: http://www.tht.org.uk/myhiv/Staying-healthy/Health-Wealth-and-Happiness (accessed 2 October 2017).

13 Carers

Figure 13.1 Cycle of discontent. Source: Jurgens *et al.* (2012). © Jurgens *et al.*, licensee BioMed Central Ltd, 2012.

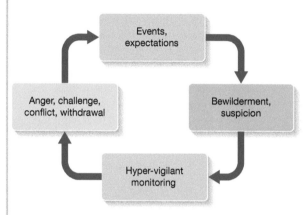

Box 13.1 Action healthcare professionals need to consider in meeting carer information needs.

- Be proactive in your information provision by establishing the most appropriate source and format for the carers you are engaged with.
- Provide verbal and written information presented in a non-technical language (font size 12 or greater for written information).
- Individualised help may be required in processing information (especially if English is not the person's first language).
- The information needs of carers change over time (e.g. in cases of stroke) and need to be proactively addressed by health professionals.
- Online information may be especially useful for carers who are socially isolated. For those without internet access, planning follow-up phone calls to assess ongoing needs may be appropriate.

Box 13.2 How to identify and support carers. Source: Adapted from Carduff *et al.* (2014).

- Include carer expert in general practices.
- Practices should ensure all new patients are asked at registration if they are or have a carer or a caring role. They can then be coded and added to a register of carers so that needs of the carer can be considered during any consultation.
- Primary care teams need to advertise more effectively the services available to carers.
- Community teams need to know what services are available and how to signpost to the most appropriate source.

Figure 13.2 An 'optimum interface'. Source: McPherson *et al.* (2014). Reproduced with permission of Elsevier.

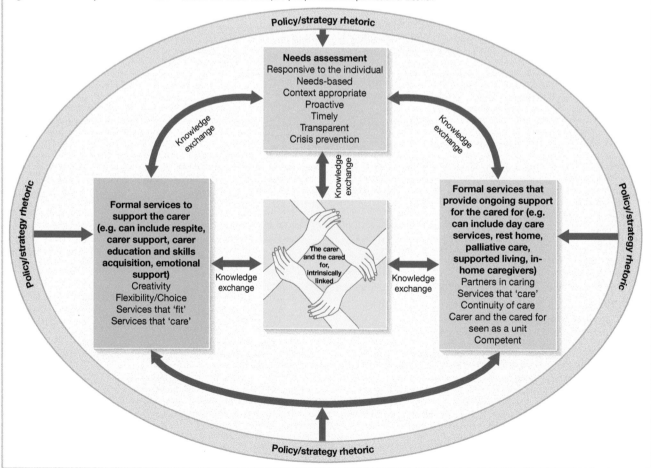

Nursing Older People at a Glance, First Edition. Edited by Josie Tetley, Nigel Cox, Kirsten Jack and Gary Witham.
© 2018 John Wiley & Sons, Ltd. Published 2018 by John Wiley & Sons, Ltd.

Carer information needs

There are 6 million informal carers in the UK and in financial terms it is estimated to save the UK economy £119 billion per year (Carers UK, 2011). One in five carers (20%) are aged between 50 and 64. In the older age range, 65% of carers between 60 and 94 years old have a long-term health issue or disability. Of the UK's carers, 42% of carers are men and 58% are women, with 1.4 million carers in the UK providing over 50 hours of unpaid care a week. There are still significant unmet needs amongst carers of older adults particularly in relation to obtaining relevant information and education to support people with chronic health conditions. In particular:

• A need for both general knowledge about disease and illness and information about the condition of the care recipient.

• A need for financial guidance and information about available services for carers.

• Carers need specific person-centred information about their care recipient especially if it is likely to impact on their identity as a carer.

Box 13.1 indicates the actions healthcare professionals need to consider in meeting carer information needs.

Carer involvement in formalised healthcare

Including carers in the management of older people with chronic conditions is an essential component of any nursing care for a number of reasons. Firstly, health professionals tend to overemphasise the significance of their impact on patients, forgetting that it is the carer who both knows the care recipient and delivers the majority of care at home. Secondly, by excluding the carer, particularly within an acute setting, mistrust and miscommunication can lead to what Jurgens et al. (2012) refer to as a 'cycle of discontent' related to concerns of quality of care and lack of control (Figure 13.1). Carers often have a clear sense of responsibility that is foundational and fundamental in nature. This can lead to hypervigilance in maintaining standards of care. Watching the standards of care and gatekeeping formal carers is common to ensure they can be trusted to deliver high quality care. The carer's needs are often met when they are certain the person they support is cared for.

Health professionals cannot practise person-centred care when they do not involve carers, and this is particularly significant in the presence of a cognitive impairment like dementia in which capacity may be compromised. Effective partnership with carers is important in patient discharge of older people, for example, in relation to medicines, creating appropriately designed written lists to supplement verbal information for carers/patients and improving communication with general practitioners and community pharmacists (Knight et al., 2011).

Hidden carers

There are challenges in supporting people who care since carers only come forward to ask for help if they recognise themselves as carers. This often occurs at crisis point since when things are going well there is often limited identification as a carer, and when supporting someone becomes very challenging seeking and navigating formalised care services can be a difficult process. The UK Care Act 2014 gives the first entitlement to support carers with an initial assessment of need (including a financial assessment if necessary) and this is mapped to the care 'journey'. There are also certain groups that remain reluctant to access care because of stigma, including carers from black and minority ethnic groups (Moriarty et al., 2011) and young carers. Three key issues influence who provides care and why and these usually centre on relationships (familial obligations), geography (siblings or friends living near the care recipient) and employment (the work capacity to have the flexibility to provide or coordinate care). Promoting carer identification is an important issue, and Box 13.2 indicates ways in which carers could be identified and supported.

Partners in care

Carers are not so much in need of care but rather a supportive partnership with service providers. This is a more meaningful and fruitful way to conceptualise the relationship. Many carers do not have any or enough opportunities to discuss the amount of caring with a health professional and when they do, a compassionate, person-centred approach is a key quality marker for carers. There is clear difficulty in both awareness of and navigating through the formal services available. Health professionals need to be proactive but are often reluctant to discuss services because resources are often limited and there is a fear of being overwhelmed by unsustainable demand. McPherson et al. (2014) propose an 'optimum interface' (Figure 13.2) highlighting the needs of carers within service provision and asserting the most important aspect for carers.

References

Carduff, E., Finucane, A., Kendall, M., Jarvis, A., Harrison, N., Greenacre, J. and Murray, S.A. (2014) Understanding the barriers to identifying carers of people with advanced illness in primary care. *BMC Family Practice* 15: 48.

Carers UK (2011) Valuing Carers 2011. Calculating the value of carers' support. Available at: http://circle.leeds.ac.uk/files/2012/08/110512-circle-carers-uk-valuing-carers.pdf (accessed 19 September 2017).

Jurgens, F.J., Clissett, P., Gladman, J.R.F. and Harwood, R.H. (2012) Why are family carers of people with dementia dissatisfied with general hospital care? A qualitative study. *BMC Geriatrics* 12: 57.

Knight, D.A., Thompson, D., Mathie, E. and Dickinson, A. (2011) 'Seamless care? Just a list would have helped!' Older people and their carer's experiences of support with medication on discharge home from hospital. *Health Expectations* 16: 277–291.

McPherson, K.M., Kayes, N.K., Moloczij, N. and Cummins, C. (2014) Improving the interface between informal carers and formal health and social services: A qualitative study. *International Journal of Nursing Studies* 51: 418–429.

Moriarty, J., Sharif, N. and Robinson, J. (2011) Black and Minority Ethnic People with Dementia and Their Access to Support and Services. SCIE Research Briefing 35. London: Social Care Institute for Excellence.

Useful contacts and organisations

AgeUK (http://www.ageuk.org.uk/home-and-care/advice-for-carers/are-you-a-carer/).

Carers Trust (www.carers.org).

Carers UK (http://www.carersuk.org).

GOV.UK. Carer's allowance (https://www.gov.uk/carers-allowance/overview).

GOV.UK. Care Act 2014 (https://www.gov.uk/government/publications/care-act-2014-part-1-factsheets).

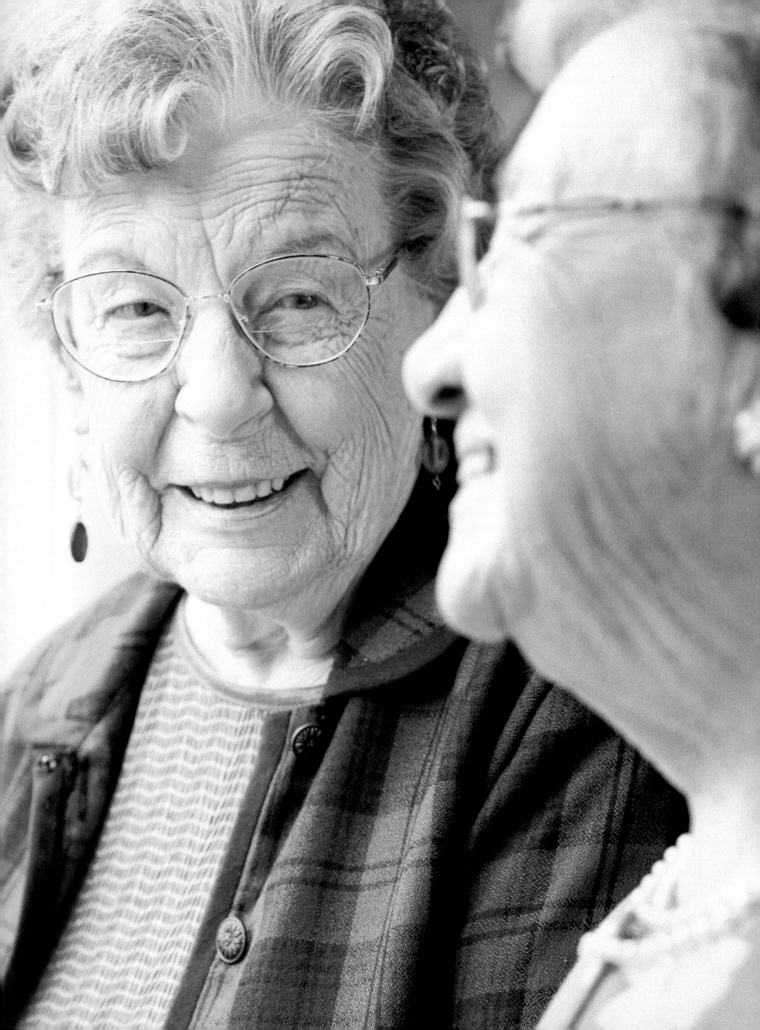

Promoting health in practice

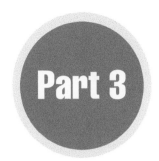

Part 3

Chapters

14 Health promotion

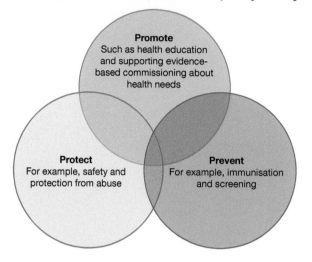

Figure 14.1 A framework for promoting health in all nursing. Source: Adapted from Royal College of Nursing (2012). Reproduced with permission of the Royal College of Nursing.

Promote
Such as health education and supporting evidence-based commissioning about health needs

Protect
For example, safety and protection from abuse

Prevent
For example, immunisation and screening

Box 14.1 Benefits of regular physical activity for older people. Source: Adapted from CMO (2011).

- Maintains bone density.
- Reduces the risk of fractures.
- Reduces the risk of falls.
- Improves mood.
- Lowers blood pressure.
- Maintain independence and social engagement.
- Reduces risk of developing dementia (Windle *et al.*, 2010).
- Increases muscle strength resulting in improvements in functional aspects of daily living amongst the older frail person (Windle *et al.*, 2010).

The ultimate goal in understanding and improving people's health is to make a difference to the causes of ill health and disease, rather than just focusing on the consequences of it. This, for nurses, can present somewhat of a challenge as they face the constraints of focusing on the causes of ill health and disease in their day-to-day work. Modern nursing should, however, involve much more than just addressing symptoms. It should concentrate on the causes and prevention of ill health rather than responding to its effects. Addressing disease prevention, promoting positive health and extending life is what

nurses do in their day-to-day work, and older people have a great deal to gain from effective health promotion. Ill health prevention is a key feature of health promotion, and the promotion of healthy lifestyles to older people is influential in helping to avoid the deterioration in health that is traditionally associated with ageing. This has been highlighted in both government and nursing documentation (Figure 14.1) (Department of Health, 2010; Royal College of Nursing, 2012). Health promotion for older people also has a central role to play in mitigating the disabling outcomes of illness amongst those who are already ill. There are three major levels of preventative health promotion:

- **Primary prevention:** This is aimed at preventing disease before it occurs. Examples for the older person may be the prevention of influenza or pneumococcal pneumonia through the annual immunisation programme.
- **Secondary prevention:** This aims to identify people at risk and prevent any further deterioration in their health and well-being. For an older person this may include screening and assessment to identify specific health conditions, which may result in further problems such as falls or injury.
- **Tertiary prevention:** This involves interventions to improve the health of somebody who already has a disease by restoring them back to their optimum level of health, minimising the negative effects of disease, and preventing further disease-related complications. In an older person this may, for example, include interventions to delay many complications related to arthritis, heart disease or diabetes.

All three preventative levels can make a difference to the health and well-being outcomes of older people. Even amongst the oldest age groups, there is potential for improving health as people get older.

Nursing and health promotion in older people

Nurses are in an ideal position to influence the people they interact with, empowering them to achieve positive health outcomes:

Whether this is by engaging in primary prevention, taking action to reduce the incidence of disease; or through secondary prevention, by systematically detecting the early stages of disease and intervening before full symptoms develop; or through good health teaching and the promotion of self-care management, it is nurses who remain a key influencing contact

Royal College of Nursing (2012, p. 2)

All nurses in primary and secondary care are well placed to promote the health and well-being of older people. We can take, for example, the benefits of participating in some form of regular exercise (Box 14.1). By modifying the intervention to suit the environment in which the older person lives and any underlying illness, nurses in both primary and secondary care settings have the potential to influence positive outcomes for the health and functional status of older people.

Falls are a major cause of disability and the leading cause of mortality resulting from injury in people aged 75 and older in the UK (NICE, 2014). The participation of older people in falls prevention programmes is a key intervention in preventing falls. Nurses have an important role to play in promoting falls prevention and facilitating older people's access to falls prevention programmes.

Making every contact count

The examples given of the benefits of exercise for older people and falls prevention programmes demonstrate how nurses can promote the health and well-being of older people in their day-to-day work. Nurses are in a unique position in relation to the

health and well-being of older patients and their carers, to Make Every Contact Count (Department of Health, 2010):

Making Every Contact Count, where timely and opportunistic advice is given in a healthcare or a community setting, is a key part of health promotion

Nursing Times (2015)

Using opportunities during nursing assessment, nursing care and hospital discharge planning to have timely 'health chats' with older patients and their carers can result in positive outcomes. Making Every Contact Count in visits to residential care homes and other work with communities offers nurses opportunities to promote healthy lifestyles and prevention strategies.

The future for health promotion in older people

Many people are not only living longer but also living full and healthy lives into older age. Health promotion programmes for older people will need to be appropriate for those who have chronic disease and those who are frail and dependent. Enabling older people with chronic diseases to adopt health protective and self-management behaviours can help them to live more independently. For nursing, there is a need to ensure that enabling and preventative approaches to health promotion for older people are fundamental for all nurses working in primary and secondary care across all settings.

Nurses in all settings are well placed to promote the health and well-being of older people. Modern nursing is more than addressing symptoms. It should work to address the causes and prevention of ill health rather than responding to its effects.

Nurses are in a unique position to implement 'Make Every Contact Count' (Department of Health, 2010) to support the health and well-being of older patients and provide support for their carers. In a society that is inevitably ageing, the key issue for nursing is that effective health promotion should be a fundamental aspect of routine nursing care.

References

CMO (Chief Medical Officers) of England, Scotland, Wales and Northern Ireland (2011) Start active, stay active: a report on physical activity from the four home countries' Chief Medical Officers. London: Department of Health, Physical Activity, Health Improvement and Protection.

Department of Health (2010) Improving the health and well-being of people with long-term conditions. World class services for people with long-term conditions – information tool for commissioners. London: HMSO.

NICE (2014) Falls: the assessment and prevention of falls in older people. National Institute for Health and Care Excellence.

Nursing Times (2015) Nurses have a major role in making every contact count. Available at: http://www.nursingtimes.net/nursing-practice/practice-comment/nurses-have-a-major-role-in-making-every-contact-count/5078261.article (accessed 19 September 2017).

Royal College of Nursing (2012) Going upstream: nursing's contribution to public health. London: RCN.

Windle, G., Hughes, D., Linck, P., Russell, I. and Woods, B. (2010) Is exercise effective in promoting mental well-being in older age? A systematic review. *Aging and Mental Health* 6: 652–669.

Falls and falls prevention in older people

Table 15.1 World total population and population aged 65 and over by sex: 2015, 2030 and 2050 (numbers in millions). Source: He *et al.* (2015).

Year	Total population			Population aged 65 and over			Percentage aged 65 and over		
	Both sexes	Male	Female	Both sexes	Male	Female	Both sexes	Male	Female
2015	7253.3	3652.0	3601.3	617.1	274.9	342.2	8.5	7.5	9.5
2030	8315.8	4176.7	4139.1	998.7	445.2	553.4	12.0	10.7	13.4
2050	9376.4	4681.7	4694.7	1565.8	698.5	867.3	16.7	14.9	18.5

Figure 15.1 Interventions for the prevention of falls. Source: Réseau francophone de prévention des traumatismes et de promotion de la sécurité under the direction of Hélène Bourdessol and Stéphanie Pin (2008). Reproduced with permission of Santé Publique France/Stéphanie Pin.

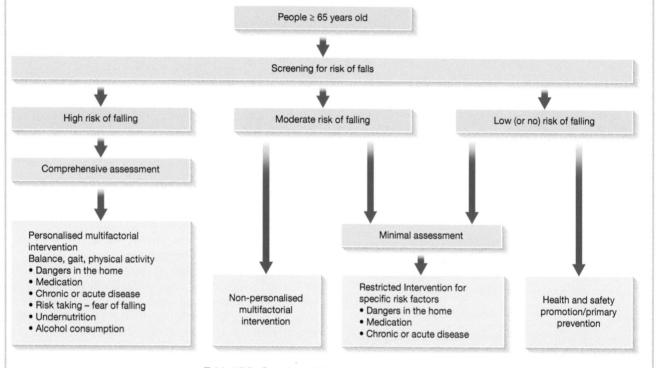

Table 15.2 Overview of the main risk factors for falls in elderly people. Source: WHO (2008). Reproduced with permission from WHO.

Category	Risk factors
Demographic	Race (being Caucasian) Low socioeconomic status
Biological	Older age Sex (being female)
Medical conditions	Diabetes Alzheimer's disease Depression Parkinson's disease Incontinence (mixed)
Physical	Poor gait/balance Previous falls Muscle weakness Low body mass index (BMI) Visual impairment Foot problems Cognitive impairment
Environmental	E.g. stairs/steps

The world population is ageing dramatically although fertility has fallen to very low levels in many parts of the world. In 2012, when the world population was nearly 7 billion, 8% were aged 65 and over. By 2015 this proportion had reached 8.5%. It is estimated that this older population will be approximately 1.6 billion by 2050 but, interestingly, the total population will increase by 34% at the same time (Table 15.1) (He *et al.*, 2015).

The frequency of falls increases with age, and this increased tendency to fall with age is a major problem for healthcare providers as well as for older people and their carers. The chance of falling increases with age, and almost one-third of older people fall each year (Bergland, 2012). Furthermore, approximately 28–35% of elderly people (aged 65 and over) fall each year, increasing to 32–42% for those aged 70 and over (WHO, 2007).

Identifying and treating the reasons for falling is very useful for prevention of falls. Fall prevention is of a multidisciplinary nature.

Description of falling

Falls are a major public health problem that lead to considerable mortality, morbidity and reduced functioning (Rose and Hernandez, 2010). A common definition of a fall is when a person inadvertently comes to rest on the ground, floor or other lower level, excluding intentional changes in position.

Types of falls

Identification of falls is very important because different types of fall have different measures for prevention. We can classify falls as accidental falls, anticipated physiological falls and unanticipated physiological falls (WHO, 2007).

• **Accidental falls:** Accidental falls are caused by patients or the reasons are due to environmental factors (WHO, 2007).

• **Anticipated falls and unanticipated falls:** Anticipated falls generally occur if a patient has been identified as fall-prone by scoring their risk of falling (WHO, 2007).

Risk factors for falls

Falls in elderly people are frequently the result of intrinsic factors or extrinsic factors. These factors can be classified into four categories: biological, behavioural, environmental and social and economic risk factors. There are also activity-related causes, that is risk-taking behaviour, such as a resident not using a prescribed walking aid. An individual can face more than one risk factor (Table 15.2).

Preventions of falls

There are many interventions for fall prevention, which can be classified into several broad categories (Figure 15.1):

• multi-dimensional fall risk assessment coupled with risk reduction;

• exercise programmes of various types;

• environmental evaluation and modification;

• multifactorial interventions;

• institutional interventions.

Even though the aim of all interventions is to prevent falls, their approach is different (Rose and Hernandez, 2010).

In addition, physical exercise programmes (which include strength and balance training) can plainly improve strength, endurance and body mechanics. Several controlled trials have shown significant reduction in falls (AGS/BGS/AAOS, 2011); exercise that was especially effective includes tai chi or the Otago Exercise Programme, balance and gait training, and strength building. Other important issues include: a balanced diet with only small quantities of alcohol; correct use of medication, especially psychotropic medications; and safety in the home (e.g. clutter, poor lighting, throw rugs, raised toilet seats – which can be addressed through home visits by an occupational therapist or home intervention team). Interventions to mitigate home dangers or risks will improve safety and have a positive effect on general health and fall prevention, and should be encouraged (NICE, 2013).

Education and information about preventing falls

Individuals at risk of falling, and their carers, should be offered information verbally in writing, about:

• What measures they can take to prevent further falls.

• How to stay motivated if referred for falls prevention strategies that include exercise or strength and balancing components.

• The preventable nature of some falls.

• The physical and psychological benefits of modifying falls risk.

• Where they can seek further advice and assistance.

• How to cope if they have a fall, including how to summon help and how to avoid a lengthy period of recumbency before help arrives (NICE, 2013).

References

AGS/BGS/AAOS Panel for the Prevention of Falls in Older Persons, American Geriatrics Society and British Geriatrics Society (2011) Survey of the updated American Geriatrics Society/British Geriatrics Society clinical practice guideline for prevention of falls in older persons. *Journal of the American Geriatrics Society* 59(1): 148–157.

Bergland, A. (2012) Fall risk factors in community-dwelling elderly people. *Norsk Epidemiologi* 22: 151–164.

He, W., Goodkind, D. and Kowal, P. (2015) *An Aging World: 2015*. U.S. Census Bureau, International Population Reports, P95/16-1. Washington, DC: U.S. Government Publishing Office.

NICE (2013) Falls in older people: assessing risk and prevention. Clinical guideline CG161. London: National Institute for Health and Care Excellence. Available at: https://www.nice.org.uk/guidance/cg161 (accessed 19 September 2017).

Réseau francophone de prévention des traumatismes et de promotion de la sécurité under the direction of Hélène Bourdessol and Stéphanie Pin (2008). *Prevention of falls in the elderly living at home*. Good Practice Guide (trans. Erwin, K.L.). Saint-Denis: INPES [original in French, 2005].

Rose, D.J. and Hernandez, D. (2010) The role of exercise in fall prevention for older adults. *Clinics in Geriatric Medicine* 26: 607–631.

WHO (2007) WHO Global report on falls prevention in older age. World Health Organization.

WHO (2008) WHO global report on falls prevention in older age. Geneva: World Health Organization.

16 Medication management

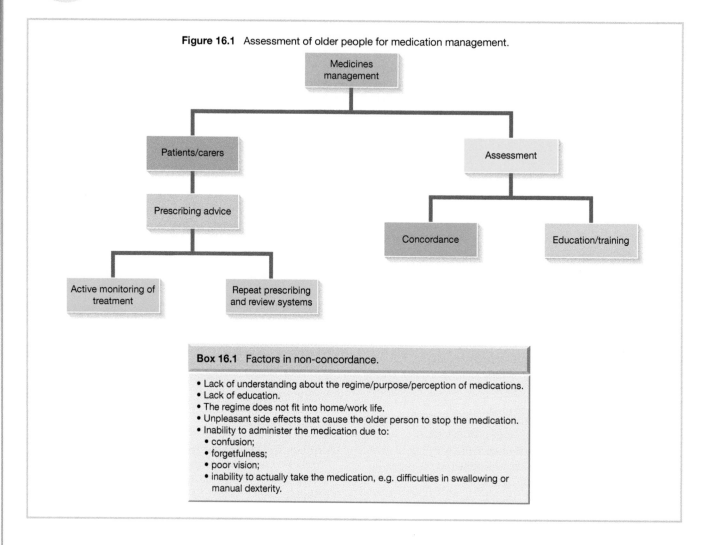

Figure 16.1 Assessment of older people for medication management.

- Medicines management
  - Patients/carers
    - Prescribing advice
      - Active monitoring of treatment
      - Repeat prescribing and review systems
  - Assessment
    - Concordance
    - Education/training

Box 16.1 Factors in non-concordance.

- Lack of understanding about the regime/purpose/perception of medications.
- Lack of education.
- The regime does not fit into home/work life.
- Unpleasant side effects that cause the older person to stop the medication.
- Inability to administer the medication due to:
  - confusion;
  - forgetfulness;
  - poor vision;
  - inability to actually take the medication, e.g. difficulties in swallowing or manual dexterity.

Medicines management

Assessment

It is essential that older people are assessed for their ability to take their own medications, with the overall aim being to enable them to be as self-caring as possible. In order to do this, discussion with the older person must include their daily activities of living, home routine, and social and, where appropriate, work life so that a medication regime can be prescribed that fits into their existing routine. Not only should a full and comprehensive medical history be taken but also a psychological assessment in order to assess the older person's ability to achieve concordance with their medication regime (Figure 16.1).

Concordance

Non-concordance in relation to medicine taking can be problematic. The majority of older people will be self-caring and able to self-administer their own medications but may require some support, particularly when dealing with multiple medications/complex regimes. Therefore, it is important that the older person is assessed for their suitability to do this. They may be non-concordant due to a number of factors, which may or may not be associated with their age (Box 16.1).

It is recognised that some older people will be taking multiple medications concurrently and that there are risks associated with this. It is important to recognise that these risks need to be managed in order for the person to gain maximum benefit from their medications and to maintain their quality and duration of life. This will also prevent unnecessary harm for the older person due to illness as a result of inappropriate or excessive administration of medicines. Side effects are often managed by prescribing additional medications, which may lead to inadvertent polypharmacy (see Chapter 17). There are a number of strategies that can be implemented for the effective and safe management of medication.

Education and training

It is essential that all parties involved in the older person's care work together, in conjunction with the older person, to maintain his or her independence and healthy life. This may include maintaining the self-administering of medication, which may require some form of support, either education or training for the older persons and carer(s). It may be necessary to involve other services in the short term to assist with the administration of medication. Ultimately, as with any adult, the goal is to self-manage.

Patients and carers

There are a number of practical methods to assist in the administration of medication. Dosette or pill boxes can be effective in achieving self-care. Patient packs of medicines are generally helpful but older people may have particular difficulties with the packaging, such as blister or foil packaging. Liaising with the pharmacist and drug representatives may be useful in order to find the most suitable formulation of drug.

Prescribing advice/support

Older people have a higher prevalence of chronic illness and are therefore more likely to be taking medication prescribed by their healthcare team. This may include multiple prescribers working independently; therefore, effective ongoing advice and support about an older person's medications is required in an attempt to reduce the risk of the recipient suffering adverse drug reactions. Ongoing communications (verbal, written and electronic) are essential amongst all prescribers and those administering medications in order to reduce any risks. This may also include any carers who are involved in the administration of medication. All those involved must be aware of what the older person is taking to reduce any drug-to-drug interactions when reviewing medications or prescribing something new. It is important to teach the older person and their carers about their multiple medications, such as the name, appearance, purpose, effects, side effects and possible drug-to-drug interactions.

Active monitoring of treatment

The goals of active monitoring of treatment are to ensure that the intended effects of the medicines are produced and remain appropriate. Routine and regular monitoring of medications should include checking whether the patient is still able to self-administer and remain independent or whether there is a need for additional support. Based on the findings, improved monitoring may be required for more effective liaisons between health and social care professionals, who play a very important role in maintaining older people's health and independence. In addition,

the older person should take responsibility in reporting and liaising with the healthcare team about managing their medication. Practical issues should be considered such as whether the older person is able to maintain independence by self-administering their medication. Providing contact numbers or helplines for the older person to call if they have any issues can be helpful. Problems that older people may encounter may include dealing with complex regimes and practical issues such as removing medicines from containers, difficulties in reading labels and forgetting to take medicines, which can be common. All these must be continually monitored and assessed in order to maintain independence.

Repeat prescribing and review systems

This group of clients require a robust and continuous review of their medication regime, which often involves the prescribing of repeat medication. It is important that the prescribing team review the older person regularly and effectively. This may include the monitoring of current medications and any additional medications such as:

• over the counter (OTC);
• herbal;
• homeopathic;
• medications purchased over the internet;
• medications given/borrowed by 'others' (such as friends, neighbours, relatives).

Ongoing review of medication is of particular importance because older people typically take more medicines due to long-term chronic illness and are more likely to take additional medications, as listed above. They are also more likely to have multiple prescribers involved in their care and are more at risk of polypharmacy issues (see Chapter 17). This not only increases the chances of unnecessary medicines being prescribed but also increases the likelihood of experiencing an adverse drug reaction. As such the dose and delivery need to be adjusted according to the age and medical/psychological condition of the older person.

Summary

The assessment, prescribing, administration and monitoring of multiple medications for older people can be problematic. Older people are more likely to have medications prescribed which are not necessary. Therefore, caring for an older person who may require multiple medications requires additional consideration from the nurse in order to reduce harm.

Further reading

Department of Health (2001) National service framework: older people. London: DoH.

Malhotra, A., Maughan, D., Ansell, J., Lehman, R., Henderson, A., Gray, M. et al. (2015) Choosing Wisely in the UK: the Academy of Medical Royal Colleges' initiative to reduce the harms of too much medicine. British Medical Journal 350: 2308.

Milton, J.C., Hill-Smith, I. and Jackson, H.D. (2008) Prescribing for older people. British Medical Journal 336: 606.

Patient website. Prescribing for the older patient. Available at: www.patient.co.uk/doctor/prescribing-for-the-older-patient (accessed 20 September 2017).

17 Polypharmacy

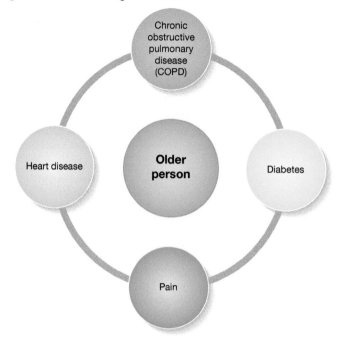

Figure 17.1 Potential long-term or chronic medical conditions.

- Chronic obstructive pulmonary disease (COPD)
- Heart disease
- Older person
- Diabetes
- Pain

Box 17.1 Problems associated with polypharmacy.

- Drugs are often prescribed that are not absolutely necessary.
- Additional drugs are often prescribed to treat side effects rather than reviewing the medication routine.
- Regimes can be complex and confusing.
- Due to the nature of some chronic and long-term conditions, many prescribers might be involved in the care of an older person.
- Older people are at risk of adverse drug reactions (ADRs) and other associated issues due to the taking of multiple medications.

Nursing Older People at a Glance, First Edition. Edited by Josie Tetley, Nigel Cox, Kirsten Jack and Gary Witham.
© 2018 John Wiley & Sons, Ltd. Published 2018 by John Wiley & Sons, Ltd.

Polypharmacy can be defined as the administration of many medications together or the use of multiple medications by one individual. Some long-term or chronic medical conditions will involve the taking of more than one medication to sustain a good quality of life and maintain a healthy lifestyle (Figure 17.1).

Polypharmacy in older people

Life expectancy has increased in the UK. Consequently more people are taking more medicines. In addition, the estimated number of people living with several long-term conditions being managed with a number of medicines will rise to nearly 3 million by 2018. It is therefore necessary to consider when caring for an older person that they may be taking multiple medications concurrently (Box 17.1).

Pharmacokinetics

Older people react differently to medications due to drug absorption rates. The drugs used to treat diseases do not necessarily change with the patient's age, but therapeutic drug levels can change as ageing alters body fat and water composition. This can cause greater concentrations of water-soluble drugs and longer half-lives of fat-soluble drugs. In addition, as the liver and kidneys degenerate with age, so to does the metabolism and elimination of many drugs. Older people can also experience a decrease in renal blood flow, reduced kidney size and changes in glomerular filtration rates. The ageing process can change hepatic blood flow and liver size, which can alter drug clearance and drug elimination.

Pharmacodynamics

Older people are often more sensitive to the effects of some medicines and consequently experience adverse drug reactions (ADRs). This is because an older person's central nervous system is more sensitive to certain agents such as opioids, anti-parkinsonian agents and non-steroidal anti-inflammatory drugs (NSAIDs), medications that often have gastrointestinal side effects.

Prevention of polypharmacy problems

The number of medications prescribed for older people should be kept to a minimum and only include essential drugs. This is particularly important with older people taking multiple medications for chronic diseases or treatments involving complex regimes. The management of the older person requiring medications is essential and often complex.

Benefits of reducing polypharmacy

There are numerous benefits in reducing polypharmacy, not just financial but also improved concordance, reduction of adverse drug reactions and improved patient outcomes. Although prescribing/taking multiple medications is sometimes necessary for older people, particularly those with long-term chronic medical conditions, prescribers and those administering medication should review the medication regime regularly, in order to re-evaluate the need for taking the medicines. If possible reduce or stop inappropriate medicines where necessary.

Many patients report a dislike of taking numerous tablets and this can lead to non-concordance. Reducing medications or stopping where appropriate can lead to better patient satisfaction. Where appropriate, non-pharmacological alternatives should be explored. As always the adverse effects of any medication should be considered against the potential benefits. Overall, the prescribing and administering of medications in the older person should be kept as simple as possible, by minimising the number of medications prescribed and any changes to medication regimes.

Summary

Older people are more likely to suffer from multiple chronic ill health due to the ageing process and as a result take multiple medications (polypharmacy). There are numerous problems associated with polypharmacy, and so reducing polypharmacy produces more benefits than harms.

Further reading

Banerjee, A., Makalu, D., Ibrahim, A., Khan, A.A. and Chan, T.F. (2011) The prevalence of polypharmacy in elderly attenders to an emergency department – a problem with a need for an effective solution. *International Journal of Emergency Medicine* 4: 22.

Department of Health (2001) National service framework: older people. London: DoH.

Duerden, M., Avery, T. and Payne, R. (2013) *Polypharmacy and Medicines Optimisation: Making it safe and sound.* London: King's Fund.

Milton, J.C. and Jackson, H.D. (2007) Inappropriate polypharmacy: reducing the burden of multiple medication. *Geriatric Medicine* 7: 514–517.

18 Skin care

Figure 18.1 Effect of ageing on skin. Source: Adapted from Peate and Nair (2015).

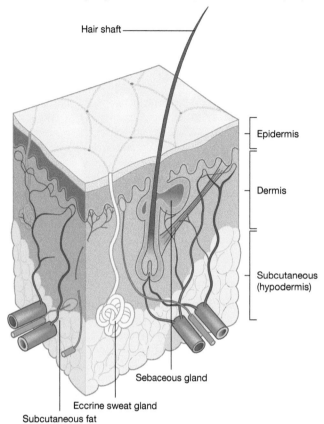

Hair shaft

Epidermis

Dermis

Subcutaneous (hypodermis)

Sebaceous gland

Eccrine sweat gland

Subcutaneous fat

Effect of ageing on skin:

Epidermis - thins, cells contain less moisture. Cell turnover rate declines. Melanocytes decrease reducing protection from UV rays. Regeneration rate varies producing lentigo senilis (age spots). Langerhans cells decrease by 50% reducing immune response. Vitamin D production decreases due to less exposure to sunlight.

Dermis - dermal epidermal layer flattens, thickness reduced. Collagen decreases and elastin fibres thicken influencing elasticity and skin quality. Greater fragility of blood vessels and decrease in numbers. Sebaceous glands produce less oil (sebum). Sweat glands decrease in number reducing perspiration and predisposing to hyperthermia.

Hypodermis - fat cell layer thins, reducing protection from trauma and insulation. Loss of fat on feet predisposes to calluses, foot pain ulceration. Nerve changes so response to pressure, pain and light touch altered.

Figure 18.2 Care of the skin in older people.

Bath/shower using warm water **not more than every second day**

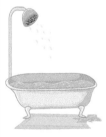

In dry atmospheres: a weekly bath/shower with daily sponge bath of underarms, perineal area and skin folds may be sufficient.
Use bath oil when 'sponge-bathing' but not in the bath or shower to avoid risk of slipping.

Use heavy creams or emollients that contain urea or lactic acid immediately after bathing. Petroleum jelly or mineral oil offer cheaper alternatives.

Pat skin dry with soft cotton towel as rubbing can damage the tissues.

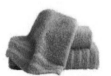

Use super-fatted soaps rather than harsh, highly scented soaps, with only one lathering.

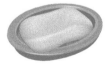

- **Avoid the use of alcohol-based rubs** or other drying rubs on the skin as it depletes the natural oils.
- Drink at least 1500–2500 mL of water a day for adequate hydration, if not contraindicated.
- Avoid tight-fitting clothes that rub the skin.

Nursing Older People at a Glance, First Edition. Edited by Josie Tetley, Nigel Cox, Kirsten Jack and Gary Witham.
© 2018 John Wiley & Sons, Ltd. Published 2018 by John Wiley & Sons, Ltd.

Looking after an older person's skin

For nurses to provide good skin care to older people it is important to understand the changes that occur as the skin ages (Figure 18.1). As a result of these changes, the external visible signs of ageing are most often seen in the skin, hair and nails of older people. However, while all skin will age, the impact of ageing processes will vary from person to person as people age at different rates. Indeed, the impacts of ageing processes on skin are determined by both intrinsic factors, such as genetic make-up, physical characteristics and hormonal balance, and extrinsic factors, including diet, medication, lifestyle choices and exposure to the sun (Cowdell and Radley, 2012). This chapter also considers the factors that contribute to good skin care for older people.

The function and structure of skin

Skin is the protective outer covering of the body and is its largest organ. Its primary function is to serve as a barrier to harmful bacteria and other threats such as pollutants and chemicals. However, skin also prevents fluid loss and dehydration, protects the body from ultraviolet rays and protects the underlying organs from injury. It plays a role in temperature regulation, via the subcutaneous fat layer that acts as insulation and as a caloric store, and blood pressure regulation due to its ability to store blood in the system. The skin also synthesises vitamin D from sunlight (UV rays), which is vital for maintenance of healthy bones (Cowdell and Radley, 2012). Hence, the skin is an important organ, and maintaining its integrity to maintain good health, prevent the risk of trauma and reduce the risk of infections is important, but this can be more difficult to achieve with ageing skin.

Ageing skin

Older people are particularly susceptible to dry skin due to age-related changes in the dermal and epidermal layers (see Figure 18.1). As a result an older person's skin can appear rough, scaly, flaky or cracked, which can indicate xerosis (dry skin). With ageing, the epidermis thins, has reduced moisture content and reduced skin cell turnover, predisposing the older person to greater trauma and also slower healing. The dermis loses about 20% of its thickness, which can result in skin appearing 'paper thin' and transparent, with fragile blood vessels that are prone to haemorrhage with mild trauma. The epidermis and dermis contact layer flattens and thus increases the fragility of the skin and also reduces nutrient transfer. Elasticity is lost and the reduction of hyaluronic acid production and sebaceous fluid output from sebaceous glands causes skin to become dry. This process starts from about the age of 40, and other contributing factors are cold weather, dry atmospheres, indoor heating and cooling systems, use of harsh, strongly perfumed soaps, astringent cleansers, frequent hot bathing or showering and bed rest (Tabloski, 2014).

Older people and skin care

As a result of changes to ageing skin, conservative care of the skin is advised as people get older (Figure 18.2). Following this guidance, bathing, washing or showering should be reduced in frequency to no more than every other day using warm, not hot water, with no excessive scrubbing. Bath oil should not be used in baths or showers due to danger of slipping, but it may be used in sponge baths in the basin. The use of a super-fatted soap is recommended, with one lathering. Other soaps may be used but only in limited amounts as harsher soaps dry the skin excessively. The skin should be patted dry using a cotton soft towel, to prevent irritation and reduce stretching/tearing of the epidermal/dermal layer. In dry atmospheres, such as centrally heated environments, one bath or shower a week may be sufficient, with daily sponge baths of underarms, perineal area and skin folds (Friedman, 2011). Older people have a decreased number of sweat glands, which means they tend to have a less distinct body odour (Miller, 2009) so the use of underarm deodorisers may be reduced as they may contain alcohol and perfumes, which dry the skin.

Application of a heavy cream or emollient is recommended, immediately following cleansing of the skin whilst it is still moist, to increase moisture retention in the skin and restore the moisture balance. Creams and emollient lotions containing urea or lactic acid are particularly beneficial; less expensive alternatives are petroleum jelly or mineral oil. The use of moisturisers on the skin should reduce the likelihood of developing skin itch. Preventing skin itch is particularly important as scratched skin offers a route for bacteria to enter the skin and cause infection.

Alcohol rubs and other drying rubs used on the skin, along with vigorous rubbing of the skin, can cause depletion of the skin's natural oils and also contribute to tearing of the cutaneous and dermal tissues, potentially causing further damage to the skin. Ensuring adequate fluid intake (of at least 1500–2500 mL of fluid a day), if not contraindicated by other medical conditions, will assist in maintaining good skin health (Freidman, 2011; Lazare, 2012).

Skin care is an important part of nursing care and it allows people to experience one of the most meaningful and powerful human senses, that of touch. Touch allows people to give and receive positive and negative messages, which are vital to remaining healthy and are a means of connecting physically to others.

References

Cowdell, F. and Radley, K. (2012) Maintaining skin health in older people. *Nursing Times* 108(49): 16–20.

Friedman, S. (2011) Integumentary function. In: Meiner, S.E. (ed.) *Gerontological Nursing*, 4th edn. Elsevier, pp. 607–639.

Lazare, J. (2012) Careful attention to aging skin. *Aging Well* 5(5): 18.

Miller, C. (2009) *Nursing for Wellness in Older Adults.* Philadelphia: Wolters Kluwer/Lippincott Williams & Wilkins.

Peate, I. and Nair, M. (2015) *Anatomy and Physiology for Nurses at a Glance.* Oxford: Wiley Blackwell.

Tabloski, P. (2014) *Gerontological Nursing*, 3rd edn. Pearson Education.

19 Pressure area care

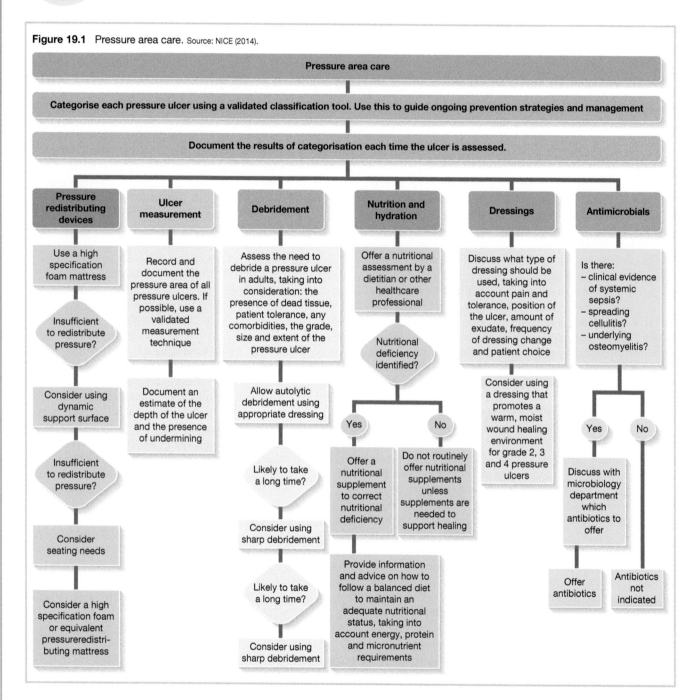

Figure 19.1 Pressure area care. Source: NICE (2014).

Assessing and preventing pressure ulcers in older people

The European Pressure Ulcer Advisory Panel (EPUAP) and National Pressure Ulcer Advisory Panel (NPUAP) (EPUAP-NPUAP, 2009) define a pressure ulcer as 'localised injury to the skin and/or underlying tissue usually over a bony prominence, as a result of pressure, or pressure in combination with shear' (p. 7). The definition identifies two key aspects: firstly, the injury or harm caused, and secondly, the cause, namely pressure or shearing. These two separate areas will be explored in relation to the care of older people.

Ahead of discussing the key aspects identified it is important to note that, although the prevalence of pressure ulcers is captured and studied when a person is cared for in an acute hospital setting, there are limited prevalence data for community care, which makes conclusions about the incidence and severity of harm difficult (Stevenson *et al.*, 2013). However, what can be ascertained is that the risk associated with developing pressure damage due to advanced age is consistent, whether in a hospital or the community. As a result of the increased risk, care strategies need to be effectively identified and deployed to reduce the likelihood and severity of harm caused to a patient

Nursing Older People at a Glance, First Edition. Edited by Josie Tetley, Nigel Cox, Kirsten Jack and Gary Witham.
© 2018 John Wiley & Sons, Ltd. Published 2018 by John Wiley & Sons, Ltd.

as a result of tissue damage through pressure. However, it is also important to note that harm caused to a person due to pressure damage is considered an adverse outcome directly attributed to the quality of care provided; most pressure ulcers are regarded as preventable if the appropriate measures had been correctly identified and implemented.

Frailty in older people and the associated risk of pressure area tissue damage

Frailty with older people comprises five criteria: weight loss, exhaustion, weakness, slow walking speed and low levels of physical activity (Campbell, 2009). These are important factors as the risk of pressure area damage increases when a person's movement is limited (Park et al., 2015). Due to the increased prevalence of frailty in the older person (Campbell, 2009), this places them at an increased risk of developing pressure area damage whether in the primary or secondary care setting (Stevenson et al., 2013). When the factors associated with frailty are cross-referenced with pressure ulcer risk assessment tools, for example the Waterlow Scale (Waterlow, 2005) or the Braden Scale (Braden and Bergstrom, 1988), the risks identified include mobility, activity and nutrition, which all serve to increase the person's risk of harm from damage to tissue from pressure or shearing. Based on this nurses must recognise and understand how frailty directly contributes to risk in an older person. Specifically in the UK, the Waterlow Scale aligns to the increased risk factors associated with older age, qualifying the individual for an elevated risk status (Waterlow, 2005). Older age increases risk along with the other elements that result in frailty. Because the risk factors for pressure ulcer damage and the factors contributing to frailty are consistent it is possible to see how the older person is highly vulnerable to pressure damage and therefore should be appropriately identified as high risk.

The importance of assessing the risk of tissue damage via the use of a validated classification tool is identified by both the National Institute for Health and Care Excellence (NICE, 2014) and the EPUAP-NPUAP (2009) as this provides a structured assessment and reassessment process to identify the risk to an individual. In particular EPUAP-NPUAP (2009) identify advanced age as a specific risk factor that should inform clinical judgement when considering an individual's risk. The frequency and validated tools used will be locally defined within organisational policy (EUAP-NPUAP, 2009). Usually the frequency of reassessment increases in response to the increase in risk. This regular reassessment should include the multidisciplinary team (MDT) to identify care strategies to prevent harm through goal setting and the agreement of a preventative plan. In addition to a regular assessment of risk a skin assessment should also be completed to ensure a structured approach is adopted, which is outlined in local policy (EPUAP-NPUAP, 2009). This will be a critical assessment to identify any tissue damage at the earliest opportunity, which should include a categorisation of the harm cause (Figure 19.1) (EPUAP-NPUAP 2009; NICE, 2014), which should then be used to inform the MDT to enable preventative and treatment strategies to be identified to address individual patient need.

Harm caused due to pressure damage to localised tissue

Categories of harm caused to tissue as a result of pressure damage are outlined in the international pressure ulcer classification system produced by EPUAP-NPUAP (2009). The classification system identifies four levels of injury, consistent with the NICE guidelines (2014):

- Category/Class I: Non-blanching erythema.
- Category/Class II: Partial-thickness skin loss.
- Category/Class III: Full-thickness skin loss.
- Category/Class IV: Full-thickness tissue loss.

For full descriptions of the classifications, please see http://www.epuap.org/wp-content/uploads/2016/10/quick-reference-guide-digital-npuap-epuap-pppia-jan2016.pdf

The level of injury is assessed to identify the harm caused as a result of pressure. Although tissue loss may not be immediately visible, clinically deep tissue injury could be suspected due to a change in skin colour (maroon or purple area of discoloration of intact skin or a blood-filled blister) (EPUAP-NPUAP, 2009). There is a likelihood that these will evolve rapidly to expose additional layers of tissue even in the presence of treatment (EPUAP-NPUAP, 2009). It is therefore imperative that any alteration to skin integrity or colour is considered significant and results in an escalation of care to obtain specialist patient assessment to inform treatment decisions by the MDT. This is consistent with the NICE guideline (NICE, 2014; Figure 19.1) as there are referral points identified to ensure specialist advice is obtained when caring for a person who has developed pressure area damage.

Validated pressure ulcer risk assessment screening tools such as the Braden scale are shown to be effective in predicting risk (Park et al., 2015); however, it is the established goals and preventative actions outlined by the MDT that decrease the prevalence and severity of pressure ulcers (Sving et al., 2014). It is therefore possible to conclude that the risk assessment is only effective as a tool if the MDT is working collaboratively to operationalise preventative processes outlined by both EPUAP-NPUAP (2009) and NICE (2014). This when applied to the older person should prompt the MDT to identify and agree a preventative plan without delay. The assessment should also be informed by a comprehensive skin assessment to identify at-risk areas of skin, which if damaged can be classified using the universal classification system. The benefit of using a universal categorisation system, standardised risk and skin assessments is consistency in communicating a patient's risk to other professionals as this will increase the promptness of the care strategies to be deployed.

References

Braden, B. and Bergstrom, N. (1988) Braden Scale for Predicting Pressure Sore Risk. Available at: http://www.in.gov/isdh/files/Braden_Scale.pdf (accessed 6 October 2017).

Campbell, K.E. (2009) A new model to identify risk factors for pressure ulcers and frailty in older adults. *Rehabilitation Nursing*, 4(6): 242–247.

EPUAP-NPUAP (2009) *Pressure Ulcer Prevention: Quick Reference Guide*. Washington, DC: European Pressure Ulcer Advisory Panel and National Pressure Ulcer Advisory Panel.

NICE (2014) *Algorithm for risk assessment, prevention and management in adults, implementing the NICE guideline on Pressure Ulcers (CG179)*. London: National Institute for Health and Care Excellence.

Park, S-H., Choi, Y-K. and Kang C-B. (2015) Predictive validity of the Braden Scale for pressure ulcer risk in hospitalised patients. *Journal of Tissue Viability* 24(3): 102–113.

Stevenson, R., Collinson, M., Henderson, V., Wilson, l., Dealey, C., McGinnis, E. et al. (2013) The prevalence of pressure ulcers in community settings: an observational study. *International Journal of Nursing Studies* 50: 1550–1557.

Sving, E., Idvall, E., Hogberg, H. and Gunningberg, L. (2014) Factors contributing to evidence-based pressure ulcer prevention: A cross-sectional study. *International Journal of Nursing Studies* 51: 717–725.

Waterlow, J. (2005) The Waterlow Score: for Hospital Community, Nursing & Residential Home Use. judy-waterlow.co.uk. Available at: http://www.judy-waterlow.co.uk/waterlow_score.htm (accessed 20 September 2017).

20 Infection control

Figure 20.1 The chain of infection.

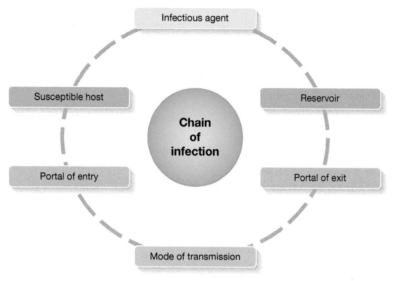

Table 20.1 Non-specific signs and symptoms of infection in older people.

Changes in behaviour	General signs and symptoms
Increased confusion	Flushed face
Reduced mobility/immobility	Urinary incontinence
Falls	Nausea
Lethargy	Cyanosis (blue discoloured skin)
Weakness	Seeking body contact
Decreased appetite/eating	Grimacing/wincing
Increased general malaise	Cough
Restlessness	Increased visits to toilet
Aggressive behaviour/angry	Red eyes
Avoiding social contact	
Anxiety	
Changed behaviour	

Nursing Older People at a Glance, First Edition. Edited by Josie Tetley, Nigel Cox, Kirsten Jack and Gary Witham.
© 2018 John Wiley & Sons, Ltd. Published 2018 by John Wiley & Sons, Ltd.

Infection is one of the ten most common causes of death in people over the age of 65 in hospital or residential care settings. Predominant infections are urinary tract infections (UTIs), respiratory infections, and skin and soft tissue infections. In older people, lack of specific signs and symptoms of infections can delay identification and treatment, increasing the risk of hospitalisation and worsening the goal of good care (Meiner, 2015).

Age-related changes to the immune system can lead to immunosenescence. This can then cause increased susceptibility to infectious diseases, decreased response to pathogens and decreased vaccine efficacy. Pera *et al.* (2015) also suggest that older people have a lower response to the split virus influenza vaccines with a consequent increased predisposition to developing influenza. Intrinsic immunity factors (thymus atrophy, bone marrow deterioration) and extrinsic factors (chronic viral infection, lack of oestrogens in older females) also influence age-associated changes in the immune response.

Nutritional and dietary status can significantly increase the risk of UTIs and respiratory infection in older people (Carlsson *et al.*, 2013), with altered taste, a physical inability to cook, altered absorption, poverty and poor dentition all contributing to inadequate nutritional status. Sjögren *et al.* (2008) show that the oral cavity is a primary source of infection for pneumonia and that mechanical oral hygiene (tooth brushing) helps to prevent older people developing lower respiratory tract infections. Tooth brushing after every meal and weekly health professional oral care significantly decrease mortality risks, and have a preventative effect on non-fatal pneumonia in dependent older people.

Psychosocial factors of stress, depression, bereavement and social relationships also have the potential to impact on older people's immune status through the role of cortisol, which suppresses the immune system, and also through a reduced neutrophil function (Vitlic *et al.*, 2014).

Lifestyle factors influence development of infection, with smoking, excessive alcohol intake, neurological disease and viral upper respiratory tract infections affecting lung function. This offers inhaled microorganisms the opportunity to survive and multiply. Social environments with multiple contact with people of all ages also increases exposure to infection.

The chain of infection

Critical to the control of infection is breaking the chain of infection (Figure 20.1). However, this is of inceased importance in older people given their altered immune responses. The chain can be broken at any point and one should consider all aspects of the chain to identify where it can be broken. For example, sources of infection (reservoir) include people's own bacterial flora (endogenous), such as *Escherichia coli* from the gastrointestinal tract, or something from their environment (exogenous), such as contaminated water or food. Susceptible people (hosts) may be those with autoimmune disease, undergoing chemotherapy or nutritionally compromised; however, genetics and other factors will affect whether the pathogens cause infection. As older people have a reduced immune function they may not show the classic signs of infection, with absence of fever, limited temperature increase and reduced or absent symptoms of pain,

The non-specific signs and symptoms that an older person may present with instead are given in Table 20.1.

Ways of reducing the risk of infection in older people

Most ways to reduce risks are simple and effective if used regularly. The principal route of cross-infection is via hands – therefore hand hygiene of all concerned is vital before and after every episode of direct contact with contaminants. Wearing of gloves is mandatory for activities that involve contact with body fluids, blood, broken skin/mucous membranes and sterile sites.

Using disposable aprons during contact with contaminated equipment or direct contact with patients prevents uniforms or clothing becoming contaminated with microorganisms. Laundry is also a source of cross-contamination; care environments will have robust policies regarding the disposal and laundering of soiled linen, which should not be carried by staff as this will contaminate their clothing. Similarly clean linen should not be carried as it may become infected from uniforms or protective aprons.

Healthcare workers are all aware of the need for 'standard precautions' in terms of infection control. These precautions become of greater importance when working with older people due to their reduced immune responses and the potential that they will also have some cognitive or physical impairment that reduces their own ability to maintain good hygiene practices.

Finally maintainence of a good diet, if necessary using supplements, to ensure optimal immune status is recommended. A fluid intake of 2000 mL per day will assist in preventing UTIs and also improve skin quality. In addition to normal bathing, care workers and patients should focus on good oral and perineal care. All should be alert for changes in smell, colour and consistency of body fluids to detect onset of infection.

References

Armstrong, K. (2015) Diagnosing and treating urinary tract infections in older people. *British Journal of Community Nursing* 20(5): 226–230.

Carlsson, M., Haglin, L., Rosendahl, E. and Gustafson, Y. (2013) Poor nutritional status in association with urinary tact infection among older people living in residential care facilities. *Journal of Nutrition, Health and Ageing* 17(2): 186–191.

Meiner, S.E. (2015) *Gerontologic Nursing*. Elsevier.

Pera, A., Campos, C., Lopez, N., Hassouneh, F., Alonso, C., Tarazona, R. and Solana, R. (2015) Immunosenescence: Implications for response to infection and vaccination in older people. *Maturitas* 82: 50–55.

Sjögren, P., Nilsoon, E., Forsell, M., Johansson, O. and Hoogstraate, J. (2008) A systematic review of the preventive effect of oral hygiene on pneumonia and respiratory tract infection in elderly people in hospitals and nursing homes. *Journal of the American Geriatric Society* 56(11): 2124–2130.

Vitlic, A., Khanfer, R., Lord, J.M., Carroll, D. and Phillips A.C. (2014) Bereavement reduces neutrophil oxidative burst only in older adults: role of the HPA axis and immunosenescence. *Immunity and Ageing* 11: 13.

21 Older people and the arts

Figure 21.1 Arts and activities for older people.

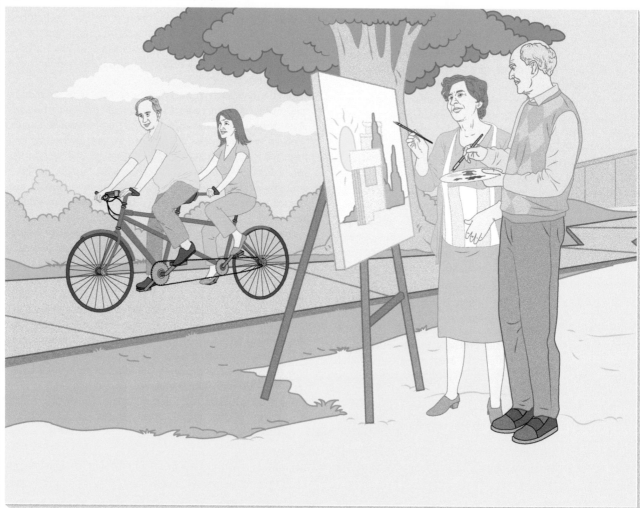

Box 21.1 The views of older people on the benefits of the arts to health. Source: Adapted from Beard (2012); Stickley *et al.* (2016).

- Improved communication with others.
- Leaving a legacy.
- Doing new things.
- Increased confidence.
- Enjoyment.
- Exploring emotions.
- Learning new skills.
- Social aspects.
- Challenging perceptions of ageing.

Box 21.2 The value of arts and culture to people and society. Source: From http://www.artscouncil.org.uk/exploring-value-arts-and-culture/value-arts-and-culture-people-and-society.

- 'Makes communities feel safer and stronger'.
- Leads to higher levels of subjective well-being.
- Attending a cultural place or event leads to good health.
- Reduces social exclusion and isolation.
- Can have a positive impact on conditions such as Parkinson's disease, dementia and depression.
- Engaging with arts and culture is associated with higher levels of subjective well-being.
- Contributes to community cohesion.
- Enriches our emotional world.
- Involvement in community arts is linked to mental well-being.

Nursing Older People at a Glance, First Edition. Edited by Josie Tetley, Nigel Cox, Kirsten Jack and Gary Witham.
© 2018 John Wiley & Sons, Ltd. Published 2018 by John Wiley & Sons, Ltd.

Background

There are currently over 15 million people aged over 60 living in the UK, and the figure is set to rise and pass the 20 million mark by 2030 (ONS, 2015). Sixty-nine percent of people aged 75 and over are living with a limiting longstanding illness (ONS, 2015). Ill health and changes in social networks can increase the risk of loneliness and social isolation, which have been linked to poor physical health and premature death. Indeed, the number of people over 50 who describe themselves as lonely has doubled since the 1940s (Victor, 2016). In order to address these issues, key priorities for improving the health of older people are now focused on active and healthy ageing, with an emphasis on prevention and health promotion. However, initiatives that aim to promote health and well-being in later life have historically tended to focus on physical activities or disease-specific interventions. In addition, traditional interventions aimed at supporting older people have not always considered a holistic model of care, for example the social aspect of ageing. Social factors need to be taken into account as across the population generally, engaging in social activities, for example, has a positive effect on self-worth and mood. One way of addressing this can be through the use of more creative and arts-based ways of working such as creative writing and poetry, which have been found to be enjoyable person-centred activities that can simultaneously benefit physical and psychological well-being and reduce symptoms in individuals with long-term conditions (Gibbons, 2012). This chapter explores a range of arts-based approaches that can be used with older people and the ways in which they can contribute to active and healthy ageing (Figure 21.1).

What are arts-based approaches?

There are many activities that could be considered when engaging with the arts such as music (e.g. singing or instrumental), writing (poetry, stories, prose), painting and drawing, drama, dancing and photography. There are advantages shown with each approach; for example, dancing has been shown to increase communication and self-reported quality of life among people living with dementia (Beard, 2012). On a one-to-one level, Higgins *et al.* (2005) explored the value of poetry reading to stroke survivors and reported multiple benefits such as relief from anxiety and an increase in emotional release, although the choice of poem was important. At a wider level, a community-based arts programme for people over 50 was shown to help the group feel more positive about their age, have increased confidence and the ability to challenge the negative stereotypes related to older people (Stickley *et al.*, 2016). The programme relied on workshops led by artists trained in various art forms such as photography, poetry and script writing. Taking part in arts-based programmes encourages older people to be part of society rather than feel excluded from it, and, furthermore, encourages the belief that older age can be a time for growth and development rather than dependency on others.

The benefits and values of an arts-based approach can be summarised as in Box 21.1 and 21.2.

Conclusion

Arts-based approaches can differ in form and style and include multiple different media. At a one-to-one or community level, benefits have been shown for physical, mental and social well-being. Considering arts-based approaches to care is important for nurses when delivering holistic care to older people. But there are many types of arts-based approaches to care for older people; approaches might be on a one-to-one basis or at a community level. Using the arts with older people promotes a positive view of ageing rather than a negative, dependent focus.

References

Arts Council England (2014) The Value of Arts and Culture to People and Society: An Evidence Review. Available at: http://www.artscouncil.org.uk/sites/default/files/download-file/Value_arts_culture_evidence_review.pdf (accessed 21 September 2017).

Beard, R.L. (2012) Art therapies and dementia care: A systematic review. *Dementia* 11: 633–656.

Gibbons, R. (2012) Writing for wellbeing and health: some personal reflections. *Journal of Holistic Health Care* 9(2): 8–11.

Higgins, M., McKevitt, C. and Wolfe, C.D.A. (2005) Reading to stroke unit patients: Perceived impact and potential of an innovative arts based therapy. *Disability and Rehabilitation* 27(22): 1391–1398.

ONS (2015) *National Population Projections for the UK, 2014-based.* London: Office for National Statistics.

Stickley, T., Hui, A., Souter, G. and Mills, D. (2016) A community arts programme for older people: an evaluation. *Mental Health and Social Inclusion* 20(1): 22–28.

Victor, C. (2016) *Summary of loneliness research.* London: Office of National Statistics. Available at: http://www.esrc.ac.uk/news-events-and-publications/news/news-items/fears-of-loneliness-in-old-age-are-largely-unfounded (accessed 2 October 2017).

22 Physical activity in older age

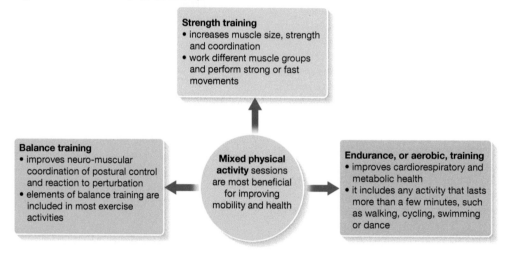

Figure 22.1 Benefits of physical activity.

Strength training
- increases muscle size, strength and coordination
- work different muscle groups and perform strong or fast movements

Balance training
- improves neuro-muscular coordination of postural control and reaction to perturbation
- elements of balance training are included in most exercise activities

Mixed physical activity sessions are most beneficial for improving mobility and health

Endurance, or aerobic, training
- improves cardiorespiratory and metabolic health
- it includes any activity that lasts more than a few minutes, such as walking, cycling, swimming or dance

Box 22.1 Exercise guidance.

- Everybody should achieve at least moderate levels of activity every day.
- Physical activity in older people has low risks of adverse health responses or injury.
- Sedentary people or those with some health concerns should gradually increase their activity over time, starting with low or moderate activities and moving to more intense activities over time.
- Separate classes should be available for people with low, medium and high capability.
- Chair-based or other appropriate bodyweight exercises are suitable for beginners and those with medical comorbidities.
- In the case of a serious adverse event, seek advice from Emergency Services.

Nursing Older People at a Glance, First Edition. Edited by Josie Tetley, Nigel Cox, Kirsten Jack and Gary Witham.
© 2018 John Wiley & Sons, Ltd. Published 2018 by John Wiley & Sons, Ltd.

Exercise for health

Physical activity, or exercise, is generally safe, and most older people do not need to consult their GP before taking up moderate-intensity activities. However, those with any concerns relating to existing conditions such as hypertension, obesity, diabetes or rheumatic problems can seek medical advice as a precaution. There are also specialist rehabilitation programmes for people recovering from more serious conditions or surgery, which are very helpful to establish the necessary underlying fitness and confidence needed to continue to exercise independently in the future. Although the benefits of regular physical activity are widely publicised and opportunities to be active are readily available, around three-quarters of older people in the UK are disinclined to exercise and instead choose to remain sedentary (Figure 22.1). The deleterious effects of sedentary living on health are at least equal to the effects of smoking, drinking excessive alcohol or obesity, and can double the risk of premature onset of ill health, disease and mortality compared to older people who are most active.

Nurses should encourage people to be more active in order to boost health and well-being. Regular physical activity reduces the risks of developing at least 26 common health conditions and can help to reduce the incidence of the most common disorders amongst older people, including: musculoskeletal conditions, which affect 14% of people aged over 65 years; heart and circulatory conditions, affecting 10%; respiratory conditions, affecting 6%; endocrine or metabolic conditions, affecting 6%; and mental disorders, affecting 4% of people aged over 65 years. Remaining active is particularly important for people entering retirement because physical activity levels tend to decline sharply and the incidence of these chronic diseases more than doubles over the following 10 years (Office for National Statistics, 2011). Regular exercise can even reverse the severity of these conditions in a dose-response manner: more activity brings greater health benefits by helping to regulate blood pressure and levels of blood cholesterol, fat and glucose. It also burns calories, which helps in efforts to control body fatness and waist circumference. Fitter people are better able to use fat taken in as part of the normal diet to make energy, rather than storing it around the major organs or experiencing prolonged periods of hyperglycaemia or hyperlipidaemia, which are risk factors for cardiovascular and metabolic disease. Regular exercise helps to maintain cognitive function and helps keep good control of movements by facilitating coordination through the neuromuscular systems, thereby contributing to reducing the risks of falling amongst older people (McPhee et al., 2016).

What types of exercise?

The general recommendations for older people are to achieve a *minimum* of 150 minutes per week of moderate-intensity activities (Box 22.1). Additionally, activities should be deliberately aimed towards increasing muscular strength and others aimed at improving balance. People are also advised to minimise the amount of time spent being sedentary – that is activities involving prolonged periods of sitting or lying.

Physical activities can be generally grouped into those aimed at improving cardiorespiratory (aerobic) fitness, such as dance, walking or jogging, and those aimed at improving muscular size and strength, such as stair climbing or lifting weights. Most common activities require a combination of strength and aerobic activities, with some components of balance training, so by being active in a number of different ways each week, older people are able to achieve the physical activity recommendations set by the international authorities.

The body quickly adapts to regular exercise and the more often a person completes a particular activity, the better they become at performing that activity, although the health and performance benefits are far-reaching and transferable to other activities. This is due to adaptations of physiological systems, most notably within the neuromuscular system to coordinate movements, the cardiopulmonary system to more effectively distribute oxygen and nutrients around the body, and metabolic processes regulating glucose and fatty acid metabolism, which collectively improve physical capability (McPhee et al., 2016).

The term *physical activity* encompasses all things that involve regular movements, such as housework, shopping, recreational walking, playing with children, organised exercise and/or sports. Organised exercise sessions need to be affordable, enjoyable, well advertised and accessible in the local neighbourhood. All of these activities involve forceful and/or quick muscle contractions, raised metabolic rate, heart rate and breathing frequency. The extent to which these different physiological systems are challenged depends upon the types of activities and the intensity at which they are performed. The intensity of exercise should be modified to best match an individual's exercise experience and physical capability, and the types of activity can be tweaked to suit personal preferences, the equipment that is available and the specific rehabilitation needs (if any have been identified).

It can be encouraging for people to be able to measure their own improvements over time. Although it does require a bit of coordinated effort, healthcare professionals or activity leaders can undertake standardised assessments to monitor physical capability and adaptations to regular training. This includes measuring walking speed over a short distance of 4 or 10 metres, or longer distances performed over 6 or 12 minutes to assess aerobic fitness. The chair-rise test gives an indication of muscular power and coordination and requires people to sit/stand from a regular chair five times as quickly as possible and the time taken is recorded, or to count how many sit/stands can be performed in 30 seconds. Balancing can be tested by asking an individual to stand with feet side-by-side, semi-tandem, tandem or on one leg for a fixed period of time (10 or 30 seconds are commonly used). To make the tests even more challenging, they can be performed with eyes closed.

When advising older people about the benefits of regular physical activity, it should be remembered that the most effective types of activities are the ones that the individual actually enjoys and will commit to completing regularly over weeks, months and years.

References

McPhee, J.S., French, D.P., Jackson, D., Nazroo, J., Pendleton, N. and Degens, H. (2016) Physical activity in older age: perspectives for healthy ageing and frailty. *Biogerontology* 17(3): 567–580.

Office for National Statistics (2011) UK General health (General Lifestyle Survey Overview – a report on the 2011 General Lifestyle Survey). Available at: http://www.ons.gov.uk/ons/dcp171776_302351.pdf (accessed 21 September 2017).

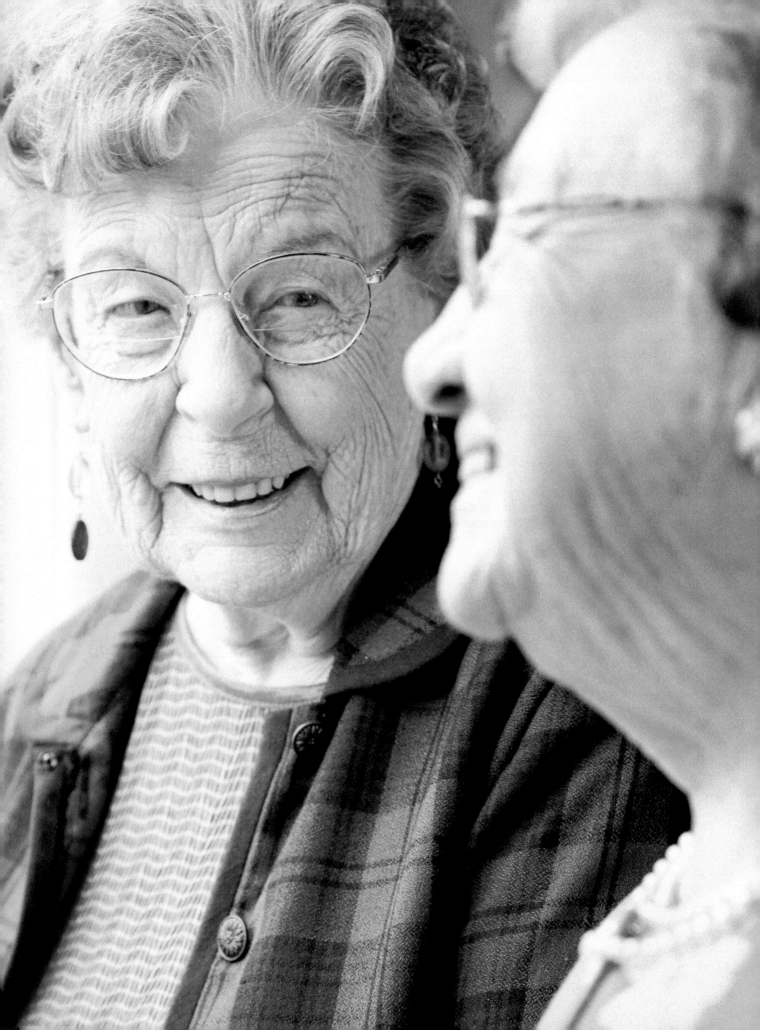

Complex care in practice

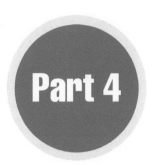

Part 4

Chapters

23 Mortality and morbidity: focus on frailty

Figure 23.1 Leading contributors to burden of disease in people aged 60 years and older – DALYs (per 1000 population) in people aged 60 years and older by cause and income region.
DALYs, disability-adjusted life years; CVD, cardiovascular and circulatory diseases; MND, mental and neurological disorders, combining the Institute of Health Metrics and Evaluation (IHME) and Global Burden of Disease (GBD) mental and behavioural disorders and neurological disorders groups.
Source: Prince *et al.* (2015). Reproduced with permission of Elsevier.

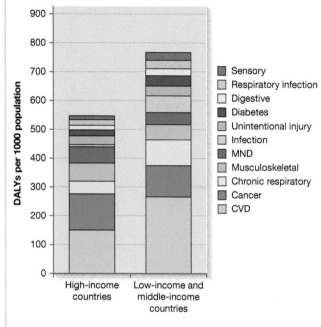

Legend:
- Sensory
- Respiratory infection
- Digestive
- Diabetes
- Unintentional injury
- Infection
- MND
- Musculoskeletal
- Chronic respiratory
- Cancer
- CVD

Figure 23.2 Schematic representation of the pathophysiology of frailty. Source: Clegg *et al.* (2013). Reproduced with permission of Elsevier.

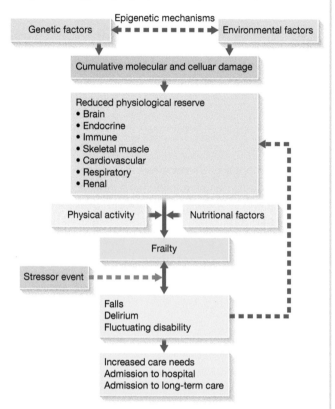

Figure 23.3 Clinical frailty scale. Source: http://geriatricresearch.medicine.dal.ca/pdf/Clinical%20Failty%20Scale.pdf (accessed June 2017). The 9-point Clinical Frailty Scale (CFS) was adapted from the 7-point scale used in the Canadian Study of Health and Aging (CMAJ 2005;173:489–495) and has been reprinted with permission of Geriatric Medicine Research, Dalhousie University, Halifax, Nova Scotia.

Clinical Frailty Scale*

1 Very Fit – People who are robust, active, energetic and motivated. These people commonly exercise regularly. They are among the fittest for their age.

2 Well – People who have **no active disease symptoms** but are less fit than category 1. Often, they exercise or are very **active occasionally,** e.g. seasonally.

3 Managing Well – People whose **medical problems are well controlled,** but are **not regularly active** beyond routine walking.

4 Vulnerable – While **not dependent** on others for daily help, often **symptoms limit activities.** A common complaint is being "slowed up", and/or being tired during the day.

5 Mildly Frail – These people often have **more evident slowing**, and need help in **high order IADLs** (finances, transportation, heavy housework, medications). Typically, mild frailty progressively impairs shopping and walking outside alone, meal preparation and housework.

6 Moderately Frail – People need help with **all outside activities** and with **keeping house.** Inside, they often have problems with stairs and need **help with bathing** and might need minimal assistance (cuing, standby) with dressing.

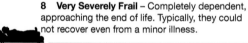

7 Severely Frail – Completely dependent for personal care, from whatever cause (physical or cognitive). Even so, they seem stable and not at high risk of dying (within ~ 6 months).

8 Very Severely Frail – Completely dependent, approaching the end of life. Typically, they could not recover even from a minor illness.

9. Terminally Ill - Approaching the end of life. This category applies to people with **a life expectancy <6 months**, who are **not otherwise evidently frail**.

Scoring frailty in people with dementia
The degree of frailty corresponds to the degree of dementia. Common **symptoms in mild dementia** include forgetting the details of a recent event, though still remembering the event itself, repeating the same question/story and social withdrawal.
In **moderate dementia**, recent memory is very impaired, even though they seemingly can remember their past life events well. They can do personal care with prompting.
In **severe dementia**, they cannot do personal care without help.

 DALHOUSIE UNIVERSITY *Inspiring Minds*

Nursing Older People at a Glance, First Edition. Edited by Josie Tetley, Nigel Cox, Kirsten Jack and Gary Witham.
© 2018 John Wiley & Sons, Ltd. Published 2018 by John Wiley & Sons, Ltd.

Frailty is a process of age-related decline in numerous physiological systems that creates vulnerability to sudden health status changes (e.g. falls) or minor stressor events. It is estimated that between a quarter and a half of people older than 85 years are frail. Frailty can be categorised as a multiply determined state of risk compared with others of the same age. It is a syndrome or a state directly related to ageing and is detectable across the life span reflecting subcellular damage. Frailty is more common amongst socially vulnerable people; both frailty and social vulnerability increase risk. Frailty leads to a greater risk of falls and it challenges health and social care in its complexity often leading to poor formalised care response. Since we all age at different rates and since this is a non-modifiable risk factor, the health provider needs to respond with a more person-centred approach.

The older people get, the more likely they are to accumulate health problems

In terms of frailty, the number of abnormal systems (e.g. the brain or immune system) is more predictive than abnormalities in any one particular system (Figure 23.1). This suggests that with the cumulative effect of multiple problems frailty becomes more of a risk. Deficit accumulation can be estimated with the frailty index:

$$\text{Frailty Index} = \frac{\text{Number of deficits in an individual}}{\text{Total number of deficits measured}}$$

The mean Frailty Index (Fried *et al.*, 2001) increases with age: the older people are, the more likely they are to have health deficits (and more of them). People of the same age have different numbers of things wrong. This is the basis of frailty. Figure 23.2 highlights the pathophysiology of frailty and the subsequent stress event that can lead to significant health problems and delayed recovery. It is important to remember that frailty as a term has a medical meaning, and using this word when talking to older people can generate negative perceptions of helplessness and weakness. Engaging with older people living with frailty and supporting interventions that may help is important rather than perceiving frailty as an irreversible consequence of older age.

Five indicators of frailty were identified by Fried *et al.* (2001); see Box 23.1.

Interventions to support frail older people

To support older frail people a number of interventions have been shown to be effective including a comprehensive geriatric assessment on hospital admission and the use of exercise to improve mobility and functional outcomes (particularly strength and balance training). Using a comprehensive geriatric assessment can predict mortality and adverse outcomes in hospitalised older patients. Interventions that used multicomponent physical training are effective, with many studies having high rates of compliance, with long duration (>5 months), performed three times per week for 30–45 minutes per session (Ng *et al.*, 2015).

Exercise is of particular importance since obesity in older life is a contributing factor for frailty especially if associated with abdominal weight gain. Issues related to mood and cognition are also important elements that need to be taken into account. Exercise has also been shown to improve emotional health in depressed older people, with physical activity potentially preserving cognitive function. A multidisciplinary approach may represent an effective approach since frailty is an accumulation of many different problems and therefore requires coordinated, longer-term management (Cameron *et al.*, 2013).

There is evidence that independently of physical exercise, nutritional supplementation may reduce frailty and increase the level of physical activity. Cognitive training programmes designed to stimulate short-term memory and improve attention, problem-solving and information processing are also effective in reducing frailty (Ng *et al.*, 2015).

References

Cameron, I.D., Fairhall, N. and Langron, C. (2013) A multi-factorial interdisciplinary intervention reduces frailty in older people: randomised trial. *BMC Medicine* 11: 65; doi: 10.1186/1741-7015-11-65.

Clegg, A., Young, J., Ilifie, S., Rikkert, M.O. and Rockwood, K. (2013) Frailty in elderly people. *Lancet* 381: 752–762.

Fried, L.P., Tangen, C.M., Walston, J., Newman, A.B., Hirsch, C., Gottdiener, J. *et al.* (2001) Frailty in older adults: evidence for a phenotype. *Journals of Gerontology Series A: Biological Sciences and Medical Sciences* 56: M146–156.

Ng, T.P., Feng, L., Nyunt, M.S.Z., Niti, M., Tan, B.Y., Chan, G. *et al.* (2015) Nutritional, physical, cognitive, and combination interventions and frailty reversal among older adults: a randomized controlled trial. *American Journal of Medicine* 128: 1225–1236.e1.

Prince, M.J., Wu, F., Guo, Y., Gutierrez Robledo, L.M., O'Donnell, M., Sullivan, R. and Yusaf, S. (2015) The burden of disease in older people and its implications for health policy and practice. *Lancet* 385: 549–562.

24 Long-term conditions and comorbidities

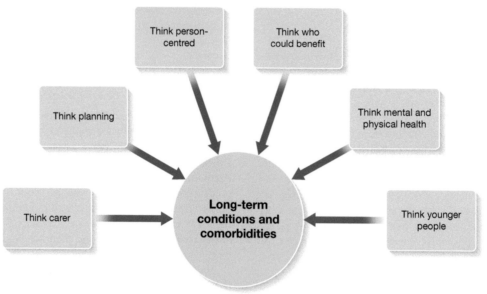

Figure 24.1 Guidance for supporting people living with long-term conditions. Source: Adapted from Moody and Bramley (2016).

- Think person-centred
- Think who could benefit
- Think planning
- Think mental and physical health
- Think carer
- **Long-term conditions and comorbidities**
- Think younger people

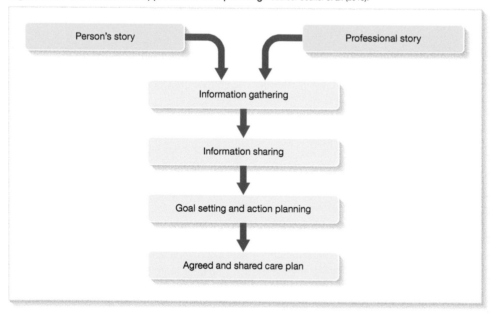

Figure 24.2 A collaborative approach to care planning. Source: Coulter *et al*. (2013).

- Person's story
- Professional story
- Information gathering
- Information sharing
- Goal setting and action planning
- Agreed and shared care plan

What are long-term conditions?

A long-term condition has been defined as 'a condition that cannot, at present, be cured but is controlled by medication and/or other treatment/therapies' (Department of Health, 2012, p. 3). Recent estimates indicate that 17.5 million people in the UK live with a long-term condition, and that this will rise to 18 million by 2025 (Saxon and Lillyman, 2011). The most common long-term conditions include: hypertension, depression, asthma, diabetes, coronary heart disease, chronic kidney disease, hypothyroidism, stroke or transient ischaemic attacks (TIAs), chronic obstructive pulmonary disease (COPD), cancer, atrial fibrillation, mental illness, heart failure, epilepsy and dementia (Department of Health, 2012; Nicol, 2015).

While understanding what the main long-term conditions are and how they are managed is important for good nursing practice, it has also been estimated that by 2018 the number of people affected by three or more conditions will be 2.9 million (Department of Health, 2012). It is therefore important for nurses

Nursing Older People at a Glance, First Edition. Edited by Josie Tetley, Nigel Cox, Kirsten Jack and Gary Witham.
© 2018 John Wiley & Sons, Ltd. Published 2018 by John Wiley & Sons, Ltd.

and other healthcare professionals to understand that the need for proactive management of long-term conditions relates not only to physical health but also mental well-being as it has been suggested that depression is seven times higher in people with two or more long-term conditions (Coulter *et al.*, 2012). However, depression is often not well diagnosed and is often untreated, which affects the abilities of older people to manage their own conditions.

Long-term conditions, whether single or multiple, can affect many parts of a person's life including their ability to work, engagement with physical activities that can make a positive contribution to health outcomes, relationships, housing options and education opportunities (Coulter *et al.*, 2012). The care and support of older people with one or more long-term conditions is also estimated to take up 70% of NHS and social care resources (Department of Health, 2012). It is therefore important that people living with long-term conditions are provided with an opportunity to positively and proactively manage their condition in partnership with a nurse or other health and social care professionals.

The role of the nurse supporting people living with long-term conditions and comorbidities

Drawing on guidance from Moody and Bramley (2016) (Figure 24.1), the Department of Health (2012) and NICE guidelines (NICE, 2016), nurses and other healthcare professionals can implement guidelines for managing long-term conditions and comorbidities in the following ways:

Think person-centred

People want to be actively involved in their care and they want to be listened to. Focus on the person, not the health conditions. Ask the person how they are managing their health. Look at what they can self-manage and what they say they need to help to manage. The collaborative approach to care planning from The King's Fund (Figure 24.2) can help guide this process.

Think who could benefit

Many people may be able to manage their long-term health conditions, but the people who are more likely to need help and support are those who:
• Find it difficult to manage their treatments or day-to-day activities.
• Receive care and support from multiple services.
• Experience both long-term physical and mental health conditions.
• Are frail or who have experienced falls.
• Frequently seek unplanned or emergency care.
• Are prescribed multiple regular medicines.

Think planning

People will be better able to manage their long-term conditions if their care is planned and takes account of:
• Proactive medication management.
• Prioritised healthcare appointments.
• Anticipated changes to a person's health and well-being.
• Someone being responsible for the coordination of care and communication with other healthcare professionals and services.
• Other areas of health, life and well-being that the person considers important.
• Arrangements for follow-up and review of decisions.

Think mental and physical health

Many people have both mental and physical healthcare needs. As noted above, people with a long-term physical condition are more likely to experience depression. People with depression are also more likely to experience poorer physical health outcomes. Assessment of both the physical and mental health of people with one or more long-term conditions is therefore important, but needs to take account of the health needs of the older person. There are many condition-specific assessment tools, and advocacy groups such as Diabetes UK, the Alzheimer's Society and the Stroke Association, along with many other online resources such as NHS Choices, publish assessment tools and can signpost people to local and national support services.

Think younger older people

Although long-term conditions are more common in people aged 65 or over, younger older people are also affected by long-term conditions. In a recent report by the Chief Medical Officer (Davies, 2016) it was reported that 7.2 million people aged 50–64 are employed, yet 42% report that they live with at least one health condition or disability. The Chief Medical Officer (Davies, 2016) also reported that these data are consistent across the UK: a study of patients registered with general practices in Scotland found that approximately 30% of people aged 50–64 have multiple physical or mental comorbidities, and 12% have both physical and mental health comorbidities. For younger older people it is therefore important that nurses take account of the need to support people who are still in employment, and pay particular attention to assessment and support of musculoskeletal conditions (21%), cardiovascular conditions (17%) and depression and anxiety (8%) (Davies, 2016).

Think carer

Moody and Bramley (2016) acknowledge that informal carers, friends and family provide considerable support to people with long-term and comorbid conditions. Nurses therefore need to take account of carers' perspectives, foster their involvement, and assess their health and well-being.

References

Coulter, A., Roberts, S. and Dixon, A. (2013) Delivering better services for people with long-term conditions: building the house of care. London: King's Fund. Available at: https://www.kingsfund.org.uk/sites/files/kf/field/field_publication_file/delivering-better-services-for-people-with-long-term-conditions.pdf (accessed 21 September 2017).

Davies, S.C. (2016) Annual Report of the Chief Medical Officer 2015, On the State of the Public's Health, Baby Boomers: Fit for the Future. London: Department of Health.

Department of Health (2012) Long Term Conditions Compendium of Information, 3rd edn. Leeds: Department of Health. Available at: https://www.gov.uk/government/uploads/system/uploads/attachment_data/file/216528/dh_134486.pdf (accessed 11 January 2017).

Moody, D. and Bramley, D. (2016) Multimorbidity – the biggest clinical challenge facing the NHS? NHS England blog. Available at: https://www.england.nhs.uk/2016/11/dawn-moody-david-bramley/ (accessed 21 September 2017).

NICE (2016) Multimorbidity: clinical assessment and management. NICE guideline NG56. National Institute for Health and Care Excellence. Available at: https://www.nice.org.uk/guidance/NG56/chapter/Recommendations (accessed 21 September 2017).

Nicol, J. (2015) *Nursing Adults with Long-Term Conditions*. London: Sage.

Saxon A. and Lillyman, S. (eds) (2011) *Developing Advanced Assessment Skills; Patients with Long Term Conditions*. Keswick: M&K Update Publishers.

25 Good practice in dementia care

Figure 25.1 Proportions of subtype of dementia. Source: Alzheimer's Society (2014).

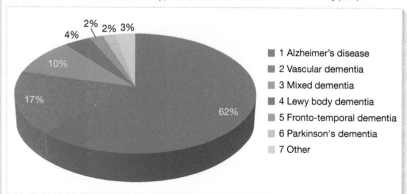

- 2%
- 2% 3%
- 4%
- 10%
- 17%
- 62%

- 1 Alzheimer's disease
- 2 Vascular dementia
- 3 Mixed dementia
- 4 Lewy body dementia
- 5 Fronto-temporal dementia
- 6 Parkinson's dementia
- 7 Other

Box 25.1   Resources for carers.

- Carers UK (http://www.carersuk.org/)
- Carers Trust (http://www.carers.org/)
- NHS Choices (http://www.nhs.uk/Conditions/ social-care-and-support-guide/Pages/carers-rights-care-act-2014.aspx)
- Dementia Friends (http://www.dementiafriends .org.uk/)
- Admiral Nurses (http://www.dementiauk.org/ what-we-do/admiral-nurses/)
- The Silver Line helpline (http://www.thesilverline .org.uk/)
- http://www.alzheimers.org.uk/site/scripts/ documents.php?categoryID=200343

Figure 25.2   Early Dementia Users Cooperative Aiming to Educate (EDUCATE).

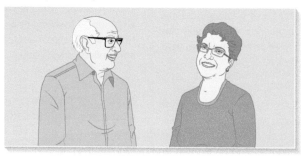

Figure 25.3   The value of patients' views – no stronger voice.

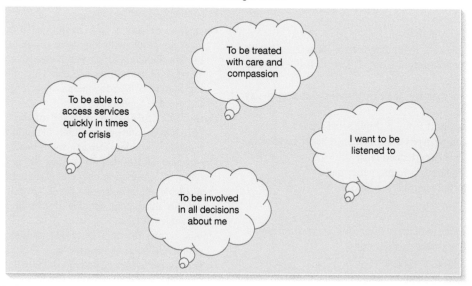

To be treated with care and compassion

To be able to access services quickly in times of crisis

I want to be listened to

To be involved in all decisions about me

Introduction

Dementia currently affects over 850,000 people in the UK (Alzheimer's Society, 2014). Despite this many people do not receive a formal diagnosis until their disease has progressed significantly. Increased public awareness of dementia was a key objective of the prime minister's challenge on dementia (Department of Health, 2015), which called for the creation of a more dementia friendly society supported by Dementia Friends. This strategy set the scene for the future direction of dementia care, aiming for the UK to be the best country in the world for dementia care. Prior to this the National Service Framework for Older People and more recently The British

Nursing Older People at a Glance, First Edition. Edited by Josie Tetley, Nigel Cox, Kirsten Jack and Gary Witham.
© 2018 John Wiley & Sons, Ltd. Published 2018 by John Wiley & Sons, Ltd.

Geriatric Society acknowledged the need for early identification, anticipation and responsiveness, together with research and support, for people with dementia, their carers and families to live well.

Types of dementia

The term dementia is used interchangeably to cover a range of specific symptoms including deterioration in cognition, functioning, mood and behaviour. The most common dementia is Alzheimer's disease, predominantly affecting short-term memory, language and reasoning. Other dementias include vascular dementia, Lewy body dementia and frontotemporal dementia (FTD). Symptoms, pathology and treatment vary significantly, resulting in the need for complex, coordinated, integrated care packages to be developed in partnership with patients, their carers and families (NICE, 2007) (Figure 25.1).

Diagnosis

Early diagnosis is essential if the difficulties and challenges faced by patients and their carers and families are to be fully met in order to deliver high-quality care and support. However, there are huge variations across the country in diagnostic rates, ranging from 30% to 80% (Alzheimer's Society, 2014). Associated fear, stigma and barriers in accessing services continue, resulting in as many as 10% of people never seeing their GP, assuming that symptoms are a natural aspect of ageing. In-depth discussions with the patient, carer and families are essential from the onset, which should also include comprehensive, advanced care planning to address physical, psychological and social needs. Dementia charities such as the Alzheimer's Society can provide a wealth of information that can help people understand the legal and ethical aspects involved in these aspects of care. However, all decision-making should be undertaken in partnership with patients and their families and should be underpinned by the Deprivation of Liberty standards and the Mental Capacity Act (Alzheimer's Society, 2015).

Referral to a local Memory Assessment Service should be the single point of referral if dementia is suspected and can provide a multiprofessional approach to diagnosis, treatment and post-diagnostic support.

Essentials of best practice: treatment and management

Dementia is a progressive illness and currently there is no cure; however, in the past decade there have been developments in this field. There are currently four drugs recommended for the treatment of dementia by NICE (2007). The aim of these drugs is to provide stability and slow progression of symptoms. However, as with all drug therapies, there are side effects and some people gain little or no benefit and this needs to be recognised. Many patients with dementia will have additional physical, mental and social needs so the diagnosis of dementia should not detract from a holistic approach to care needs. Comorbidities and contraindications need to be managed effectively, and in the early stages close monitoring is essential to identify unacceptable side effects. Carers have highlighted that this aspect of care can be the most challenging and difficult to manage so information and support is essential (Box 25.1).

Health promotion, education and health protection are essential components of a holistic approach to care. Patients with dementia should not be excluded from programmes purely on the basis of age, their diagnosis or disability without full and frank discussions with the individual and the multiprofessional team. Programmes such as the NHS Health Check also provide healthcare professionals with an opportunity to engage the patient, carers and family in healthy interventions.

Ongoing support

Projects such as the Early Dementia Users Co-operative Aiming to Educate (EDUCATE), engage and support individuals living with dementia (Figure 25.2). EDUCATE (http://www.educatestockport.org.uk/what-we-do/) focuses on the patients' perspective and develops strong alliances across health and social care to actively engage with service users. Dementia strategies for policy and practice that promote living well with dementia emphasise the importance of activities such as peer support groups.

The King's Fund (2015) identified ten key priorities for commissioners, all of which are essential drivers to improve the quality of dementia care and support. These King's Fund recommendations are focused on: systematic and proactive management of chronic disease; the empowerment of patients; a focus on the needs of the wider population (not just people who present at healthcare services); and integrated models of care. Fundamental to achieving these aims is the need to work collaboratively with health and social care including the voluntary sector and charities.

Conclusion

The number of people with dementia continues to increase; therefore future developments need patient and public participation, which helps gain insight into the experiences and views of patients and their carers (Figure 25.3).

Improved, multiprofessional training across health and social care is essential and commissioners should set priorities for ensuring frontline clinical staff have the skills and knowledge to care for the complex needs of patients with dementia. Carers are often integral to identifying early difficulties, and having good access to an integrated primary care team will avoid unnecessary crises and admission to hospital, ensuring patients with dementia are supported to live well.

References

Alzheimer's Society (2014) Dementia UK – Update. London: Alzheimer's Society. Available at: alzheimers.org.uk/dementiauk (accessed 21 September 2017).

Alzheimer's Society (2015) Mental Capacity Act 2005 – factsheet. London: Alzheimer's Society. Available at: https://www.alzheimers.org.uk/site/scripts/download_info.php?fileID=2646 (accessed 21 September 2017).

Department of Health (2015) Prime Minister's Challenge on Dementia 2020. London: DoH.

King's Fund (2015) Transforming our Health Care System, revised edition. London: The King's Fund. Available at: https://www.kingsfund.org.uk/sites/files/kf/field/field_publication_file/10PrioritiesFinal2.pdf (accessed 21 September 2017).

NICE (2007) Dementia: supporting people with dementia and their carers in health and social care. Clinical Guideline CG42. London: National Institute for Health and Care Excellence. Available at: http://www.nice.org.uk/guidance/cg42/evidence (accessed 21 September 2017).

26 Caring for the older person with delirium

Key points

1 The older person with delirium needs rapid and coordinated medical management supported by nursing care.
2 At the core of nursing care is a compassionate understanding that the experience of delirium can lead to distress and this comes through in unusual or challenging behaviours.
3 Nursing interventions help reduce distress and support the person and family through the experience until medical treatment is effective.

Nursing Older People at a Glance, First Edition. Edited by Josie Tetley, Nigel Cox, Kirsten Jack and Gary Witham.
© 2018 John Wiley & Sons, Ltd. Published 2018 by John Wiley & Sons, Ltd.

Experiencing delirium

You will encounter older people with delirium across a range of care settings, from the community to accident and emergency, medical assessment, surgical, orthopaedic and intensive care. The experience for the older person and family is disturbing and often distressing, and with many older people their distress comes out in some behaviours that may be referred to as 'challenging' for nurses, other healthcare team members and family members to respond to. A sympathetic presence is part of a person-centred response and protecting the person's dignity and privacy. At some points the older person may be aware they are behaving differently or that they are unwell and then they might become unaware of this and say and do things that are not usual for them.

Essential nursing interventions include:

- Ensuring medical colleagues respond to a delirium as a medical emergency and that a plan of treatment is in place within 2 hours (Healthcare Improvement Scotland, 2014).
- Try to get a person well known to the older person to stay with them.
- Provide sensory aids.
- Manage environmental stimulation such as noise and light.
- Use gentle orientation cues for the person.
- Assess and treat pain (Abbey Pain Scale).
- Help the person to drink and eat if they can safely swallow.
- Support family and other patients.
- Help family members to understand.

The older person with delirium may:

- appear agitated or much quieter than usual;
- be disorientated about the date, time and place;
- use different language including words they may find offensive;
- be unable to pay attention or follow directions;
- see and hear things that are not there;
- be more or less emotional than usual;
- have changes in sleep pattern;
- engage in repetitive movements and actions like tremors or picking at clothes;
- be very forgetful;
- be verbally and/or physically aggressive.

It is vital not to agitate the person so the use of restraint, antipsychotic medications and confrontation is to be avoided. This may, however, mean that some risks are increased, such as falling and skin injury.

The ABC of behaviours

To help you consider what environmental factors might influence behaviours, to understand more about the behaviour and its consequences, the ABC method can be a useful tool:

Antecedents (triggers)	Behaviour	Consequences

A behaviour occurs in response to an antecedent event or factors and generates a consequence. If the consequence is inappropriately managed, the behaviour may escalate and in turn become another trigger or antecedent. Think TIME (Healthcare Improvement Scotland, 2016):

- **Triggers**
- **Investigations**
- **Management**
- **Engagement**

TIME matters: people who develop delirium may need to stay longer in hospital, have more hospital-acquired complications, such as falls and pressure ulcers, are more likely to be admitted to nursing home care from hospital, and are more likely to die (NICE, 2010).

Recognising delirium

It is important to recognise and screen for delirium (Box 26.1). Delirium comes on quickly, in hours or days, although the signs of delirium can change from hour to hour or over a day. When it is happening, delirium causes people to experience a deterioration in their memory and thinking abilities compared to how they usually are. The course of delirium fluctuates but usually clears up after a few days or even a week providing medical treatment is provided. However, there can also be some residual effects, whereby the older person might have some thinking problems that persist for several months. At present, we do not know which older people will have residual effects and for how long.

Delirium describes a severe disturbance in cognitive and mental abilities and is sometimes called an acute confusion state. Older people with delirium are unable to think clearly, pay attention or concentrate, or understand what is going on around them in their environment; they may also see and hear things that other people do not (visual and auditory hallucinations). It is important to realise that whatever the person sees and hears feels very real to them.

Delirium is caused by a change in the way the brain functions. This may be due to multiple reasons such as less oxygen available to brain cells and tissue, an inability by the brain to use oxygen that is present, or a build-up of toxic chemicals in the brain cells. This is caused by any of a wide range of triggers including: dehydration and electrolyte imbalance, urinary retention, constipation, side effects of certain medicines (e.g. sedatives or tranquilisers), infection that the brain cannot cope with, severe pain, high blood sugar level, excess alcohol and/or other toxic substances, or withdrawal from alcohol and substance misuse. From this list it can be seen why so many older people are at risk of delirium. It is estimated that approximately 30% of older people in medical wards will develop a delirium, with this figure rising in surgical settings.

References

Chan, P.K.Y. (2011) Clarifying the confusion about confusion: Current practices in managing geriatric delirium. *British Columbia Medical Journal* 53: 409–415.

Healthcare Improvement Scotland (2016) Improving the care for older people. Delirium toolkit. Available at: http://www.healthcareimprovementscotland.org/our_work/person-centred_care/opac_improvement_programme/delirium_toolkit.aspx (accessed 21 September 2017).

NICE (2010) Delirium diagnosis, prevention and management. Clinical guideline 103. National Institute for Health and Clinical Excellence. Available at: http://guidance.nice.org.uk/CG103 (accessed 21 September 2017).

Further learning resources

Johns Hopkins Medicine. Geriatric Workforce Enhancement Program. Module 1 – Delirium. Available at: http://m.hopkinsmedicine.org/gec/nursing_education/Module_1_Delirium (accessed 21 September 2017).

27 Severe and enduring mental health problems in older life

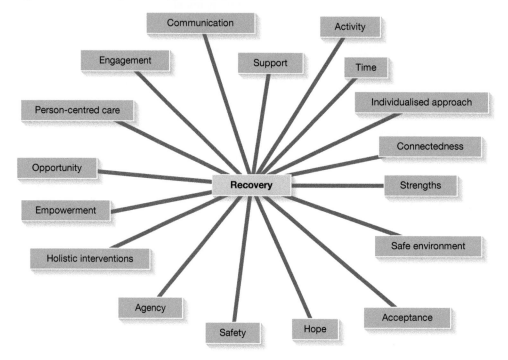

Figure 27.1 'Recovery Model' approach to care intervention.

Communication

Activity

Engagement

Support

Time

Person-centred care

Individualised approach

Connectedness

Opportunity

Recovery

Strengths

Empowerment

Safe environment

Holistic interventions

Agency

Acceptance

Safety

Hope

Box 27.1 Common signs and symptoms of severe depression.

- Low mood and sadness.
- Social withdrawal.
- Feelings of worthlessness.
- Irritability.
- Crying spells.
- Lack of appetite.
- Restlessness.
- Sleep disturbance.
- Lack of concentration.
- Confusion.
- Lack of motivation/hope/confidence.
- Thoughts of self-harm and suicide.

Box 27.2 Common signs and symptoms of schizophrenia.

- **Social withdrawal.**
- **Disorganised and bizarre behaviour.**
- **Negative symptoms** – absence of normal behaviours.
- **Delusions** – beliefs held with complete conviction, even though they are based on a mistaken, strange or unrealistic interpretation.
- **Hallucinations** – a person experiences a sensation (of touch, sight, smell, taste, and hearing) but there is nothing or nobody to account for it.

Box 27.3 The core components of the recovery approach to care.

1 **Agency** – encouraging the individual to gain a sense of control over their life and illness. Finding personal meaning – an identity that incorporates illness, but retains a positive sense of self.
2 **Creating opportunity** – building a life beyond illness. Using non-mental health agencies, informal supports and natural social networks to achieve integration and social inclusion.
3 **Instilling hope** – believing that one should still pursue one's own hopes and self-goals, even with the continuing presence of illness. Not settling for less, i.e. the reduced expectations of others.

Nursing Older People at a Glance, First Edition. Edited by Josie Tetley, Nigel Cox, Kirsten Jack and Gary Witham.
© 2018 John Wiley & Sons, Ltd. Published 2018 by John Wiley & Sons, Ltd.

Three million older people in the UK experience symptoms of severe and enduring mental health problems, which impact significantly on their quality of life. The range of such mental health problems includes depression, anxiety, acute confusion, dementia and schizophrenia. Defining the term 'severe and enduring mental health' has proved problematic over the years; however, core to all definitions is the recognition that:

1 The mental illness diagnosed has persisted for at least a year.
2 The condition has caused sufficiently severe disability to impair seriously the functioning or role performance in at least one of the following areas: occupation, family responsibilities, accommodation (Kelly et al., 2001).

Five key issues that impact on the mental well-being of older persons living with severe and enduring mental illness are:

• discrimination and stigma;
• participation in meaningful activities;
• relationships;
• physical health;
• poverty.

In older life the increased propensity for physical morbidity, in conjunction with living with mental illness, is evidenced to be extremely disabling; resulting in poor quality of life, isolation, exclusion and decreased life expectancy (Kelly et al., 2001). This chapter will consider the severe and enduring mental health conditions of severe depression and schizophrenia.

Severe depression

Approximately 1.6 million older people in the UK meet the clinical criteria for a formal diagnosis of depression (Gottfries, 2001). Severe depression is long-lasting and significantly interferes with thoughts, behaviour, mood, activity and physical health (Box 27.1).

Schizophrenia

There are approximately 70,000 older people with schizophrenia in the UK (Berry and Barrowclough, 2009). Individuals with schizophrenia can sometimes find it difficult to distinguish between what is real and unreal. It may be difficult to think clearly, manage emotions, relate to others and deal with everyday life (Box 27.2).

Approach to care intervention

Antipsychotic medication for schizophrenia, and antidepressants/ talking therapies for depression play a crucial role within care intervention packages for both conditions. However, it has been evidenced that sustained positive outcomes for individuals are enhanced when prescribed medication is used in combination with the recovery approach to care. This approach is deemed vital when facilitating the older person to manage living with severe and enduring mental illness.

Health professionals and carers committed to working from this paradigm need to accept that it is a long-term process of engagement and empowerment. This endeavours to assist the individual to optimise life opportunities and achieve their potential, through maintaining their independence, autonomy and connectedness with others.

Recovery emphasises that, while individuals may not have full control over their symptoms, they can have full control over their lives. Recovery is not about 'getting rid' of problems. It is about seeing beyond a person's mental health issues, recognising and fostering their abilities, interests and self-goals (Figure 27.1).

Mental illness, associated stigma and social attitudes to mental illness often impose limits on people experiencing ill health. Health professionals, friends and families can be overly protective or pessimistic about what someone with a mental health problem will be able to achieve. Recovery is about looking beyond those limits to help people achieve their own goals and aspirations. The process is seen as a journey rather than a destination, which requires a well-organised system of support from family, friends or professionals, calling for pragmatic optimism and long-term commitment from all concerned.

Research has found that important factors for optimising recovery include:

• Good relationships.
• Financial security.
• Satisfying work/hobbies.
• The right living environment.
• The development of one's own cultural or spiritual perspectives.
• Helping the individual (and meaningful others) to be aware of triggers for illness, and the development of resilience coping strategies.

Further factors (Shepherd et al., 2014) highlighted by individuals as supporting them on their recovery journey include:

• Being believed in.
• Being listened to and understood.
• Others maintaining a positive attitude.
• Getting informed explanations for problems or experiences.
• Having the opportunity to temporarily resign responsibility during periods of crisis.

Employing good communication and interpersonal skills, and the development of the therapeutic relationship, is always desirable when working with individuals accessing health services. However, in the case of those living with severe and enduring mental illness it is crucial, as promoting well-being and enhancing quality of life are dependent on the development of such relationships. The recovery approach requires a mind shift for professionals, where working with the individual is key as opposed to doing for. Self-autonomy, self-voice and engagement in all aspects of care should be actively endorsed by all involved in supporting and facilitating care (Box 27.3).

References

Berry, K. and Barrowclough, C. (2009) The needs of older adults with schizophrenia. Implications for psychological interventions. *Clinical Psychology Review* 29: 68–76.

Gottfries, C.G. (2001) Late life depression. *European Archives of Psychiatry and Clinical Neuroscience* 25(2): 73–79.

Kelly, S., Mckenna, H., Paraook, K. and Dusoir, A. (2001) The relationship between involvement in activities and quality of life for people with severe and enduring mental illness. *Journal of Psychiatric and Mental Health Nursing* 8: 139–146.

Shepherd, G., Boardman, J., Rinaldi, M. and Roberts, G. (2014) Supporting recovery in mental health services: quality and outcomes. Available at: https://www.centreformentalhealth.org.uk/ recovery-quality-and-outcomes (accessed 6 October 2017).

28 Recognising dying

Figure 28.1 Supportive and Palliative Care Indicator.

Does this patient have an advanced long-term condition, a new diagnosis of a progressive life-limiting illness or both?

Yes

Would you be surprised if this patient died in the next 6–12 months?

No

Look for one or more general clinical indicators:
Performance status poor (limited self-care, in bed or chair 50% of the day)
Progressive weight loss (>10%) over the past 6 months
Two or more unplanned admissions in the past 6 months
Patient is in a nursing care home/continuing care unit or needs more care at home

Now look for two or more disease indicators, for example, in dementia it may be recurrent febrile episodes, aspiration pneumonia or increasing eating problems. In heart disease it may be breathlessness or chest pain at rest or on minimal exertion, cardiac cachexia or persistent symptoms despite optimal tolerated therapy.

Box 28.1 Communication skills – being PREPARED. Source: Adapted from Clayton *et al.* (2007).

P – prepare for the discussion
R – relate to the person
E – elicit patient and carer preferences
P – provide information
A – acknowledge emotions and concerns
R – realistic hope
E – encourage questions
D – document

Box 28.2 Barriers to advanced care planning.

- The reluctance of family members to discuss end of life care.
- Passive expectation from the patient that 'someone else will decide'.
- Significant uncertainty concerning future illness and decline.
- Whether the patient accepts dying as a likely outcome.
- The patient's personal experiences and fears concerning death and dying.
- The healthcare professional's ability to engage and sustain end of life conversations.

Figure 28.2 End of life pathway. Source: Department of Health. End of Life Care Strategy (July 2008). Contains public sector information licensed under the Open Government Licence v3.0.

Step 1	Step 2	Step 3	Step 4	Step 5	Step 6
Discussions as the end of life approaches	Assessment, care planning and review	Coordination of care	Delivery of high quality services in different settings	Care in the last days of life	Care after death
• Open, honest communication • Identifying triggers for discussion	• Agreed care plan and regular review of needs and preferences • Assessing needs of carers	• Strategic coordination • Coordination of individual patient care • Rapid response services	• High quality care provision in all settings • Acute hospitals, community, care homes, extra care housing, hospices, community hospitals, prisons, secure hostels • Ambulance services	• Identification of the dying phase • Review of needs and preferences for place of death • Support for both patient and care • Recognition of wishes regarding resuscitation and organ donation	• Recognition that end of life care does not stop at point of death • Timely verification and certification of death or referral to coroner • Care and support of care and family, including emotional and practical bereavement support

Spiritual care services

Support for carers and families

Information for patients and carers

Nursing Older People at a Glance, First Edition. Edited by Josie Tetley, Nigel Cox, Kirsten Jack and Gary Witham.
© 2018 John Wiley & Sons, Ltd. Published 2018 by John Wiley & Sons, Ltd.

Good integrated and coordinated palliative care for patients in later life is dependent on health professionals recognising dying. This can be challenging in an ageing population where comorbidities are high and chronic conditions can sometimes mask the dying process. In acute care this is particularly a feature where a focus may be on curative treatment and where negative staff attitudes to older people may be evident (Gardiner *et al.*, 2011). Accessing appropriate end of life services is a key issue in order to maintain autonomy, choice and dignity in dying. Within primary care in the UK, the Gold Standards Framework (GSF) was developed in 2000 to improve palliative care in primary care by utilising a systematic evidence-based approach to optimising care for all patients approaching the end of life. Although over 90% of UK GP practices now have a register of patients nearing the end of life these registers do not capture all this population of patients. Only 27% of all patients who die are included in the register before death, with the majority having cancer (Thomas *et al.*, 2012). Since only 25% of patient deaths are from malignant disease this would suggest that other patient groups appear to be under-represented in registered end of life care. The need to address and recognise dying in a wider variety of non-malignant chronic conditions is therefore a key concern for health professionals. Recognising this need the Supportive and Palliative Care Indicator tool (Boyd and Murray, 2010) (Figure 28.1) can be a useful guide to support an assessment related to prognosis and end of life care, particularly with frail older people, as Nicholson *et al.* (2012) comment:

> the transition from 'keeping going' to 'letting go' appeared difficult to make particularly for this cohort whose resilience had perhaps kept them alive into late old age [p. 1430]

For nurses to then support and implement care for older people who are at the end of their life, there is a need to be able to discuss issues such as preferred place of care and advance directives as these are key to good palliative care.

Advanced care planning

Facilitating end of life discussions with patients is an essential element of the End of Life Care Strategy (Department of Health, 2008) but this remains challenging for health professionals. The fear of upsetting patients, being confronted with answering emotionally difficult questions, a lack of confidence in initiating and maintaining conversations and lack of certainty about prognostic indicators often leads to blocking behaviours by health professionals. There are clinical guidelines available to support health professionals in communicating end of life issues with patients (Box 28.1).

The impact of avoiding such discussions can result in inappropriate admission to the emergency department at the end of life. Indeed, evidence suggests only a minority of older patients who die with palliative care needs in the emergency department are known to palliative care services (Beynon *et al.*, 2011). Being able to help older people with advanced care planning at the end of their life is important as this is part of the national end of life care pathway. The NICE quality standard for end of life care for adults (QS13; NICE, 2011) also reinforces the importance of a comprehensive holistic assessment incorporating a personalised care plan (Figure 28.2 gives the full pathway). The barriers, however, to implementing this in relation to older people are shown in Box 28.2.

Preferred place of care

Sustaining connections and routines within the home is an important issue, particularly for the frail older person who may become more socially isolated and physically weak. Most surveys show an overwhelming preference for people to die at home although some older people acknowledge this may not always be possible, but stress the importance of the presence of friends and family at the end of life. It is therefore important for health professionals to facilitate preferences in terms of place of care and create an environment conducive to the presence of family and friends at the end of life.

It is important to address issues related to preferred place of care early on from diagnosis since certain diseases such as dementia can lead to a loss of capacity and would require a best interests assessment if choices were not established at the appropriate time. While pathways and end of life frameworks can help with care planning, it is important to understand that rigid application of pathways and care plans may fail to address the problems related to care of the dying older patient. Healthcare professionals must then also recognise that older people who are dying will need support and space to continue to live their everyday lives and build relationship underpinned by principles and values that include living well at the end of life.

References

Beynon, T., Gomes, B., Murtagh, F.E.M., Glucksman, E., Parfitt, A., Burman, R. et al. (2011) How common are palliative care needs among older people who die in the emergency department? *BMJ Supportive Palliative Care* 1: 184–188.

Boyd, K. and Murray, S.A. (2010) Recognising and managing key transitions in end of life care. *British Medical Journal* 341: c4863.

Clayton, J., Hancock, K., Butow, P., Tattersall, M. and Currow, D. (2007) Clinical practice guidelines for communicating prognosis and end-of-life issues with adults in the advanced stages of a life-limiting illness, and their caregivers. *Medical Journal of Australia* 186(12): S77–S108.

Department of Health (2008) End of Life Care Strategy. Available at: https://www.gov.uk/government/uploads/system/uploads/attachment_data/file/136431/End_of_life_strategy.pdf (accessed October 2017).

Gardiner, C., Cobb, M., Gott, M. and Ingleton, C. (2011) Barriers to providing palliative care for older people in acute hospitals. *Age and Ageing* 40(2): 233–238.

NICE (2011) End of life care for adults (QS13). London: National Institute for Health and Care Excellence.

Nicholson, C., Meyer, J., Flatley, M., Holman, C. and Lowton, K. (2012) Living on the margin: understanding the experience of living and dying with frailty in old age. *Social Science & Medicine* 75: 1426–1432.

Thomas, K., Corner, H. and Stobbart-Rowlands, M. (2012) National primary care audit in end of life care and ACP and recommendations for improvement. *BMJ Supportive & Palliative Care* 2: 192.

29 Grief, loss and bereavement

Box 29.1 Definitions.

- **Bereavement** is the process of losing a close relationship, a change in status.
- **Grief** is the pain and suffering experienced after loss, the psychological response to loss (anger, indifference, 'dissociative flight', unable/unwilling to grieve).
- **Loss** is the state of being deprived of, or being without, something one has had.
- **Mourning** is the period of time during which signs of grief are made visible.

Box 29.2 Models of grief, loss and bereavement.

- Stage and phase theories.
- Tasks for the bereaved.
- Continuing bonds.
- Dual process model.

Box 29.3 Kübler-Ross five-stage model of grief. Source: Adapted from Kübler-Ross (1975).

- Denial – No, not me.
- Rage and anger – Why me?!
- Bargaining – Yes, me, but….
- Depression – Yes, me.
- Acceptance – My time is very close now and it's all alright.

Box 29.4 Worden's tasks for the bereaved. Source: Worden (2010).

1 Accept the reality of the loss.
2 Process the pain of grief.
3 Adjust to the new situation and a world without the deceased.
4 Find an enduring connection with the deceased whilst investing in new relationships.

Box 29.5 Factors affecting the experience of grief. Source: Kinghorn and Duncan (2005).

- Age.
- Personality.
- Nature of the relationship with the deceased person.
- Culture.
- Sexuality.
- Gender.
- Levels of social support.
- Health.
- Nature of death.

Box 29.6 Complicated grief. Source: Worden (2010).

- **Chronic grief reactions** – prolonged or protracted grief, no resolution or diminishment for 12 months.
- **Delayed grief reactions** – absence of separation distress, affects subsequent losses.
- **Exaggerated grief reactions** – depression, anxiety, post-traumatic stress disorder, panic attacks.
- **Masked grief reactions** – lack of awareness that grief is the cause of maladaptive behaviour.

Figure 29.1 Stroebe and Schut Dual Process Model. Source: Stroebe and Schut (1999). Reproduced with permission of Taylor & Francis.

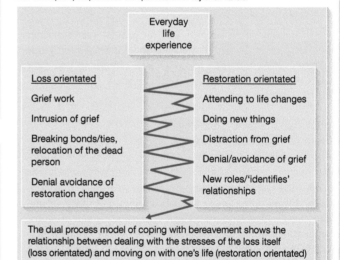

The dual process model of coping with bereavement shows the relationship between dealing with the stresses of the loss itself (loss orientated) and moving on with one's life (restoration orientated)

Nursing Older People at a Glance, First Edition. Edited by Josie Tetley, Nigel Cox, Kirsten Jack and Gary Witham.
© 2018 John Wiley & Sons, Ltd. Published 2018 by John Wiley & Sons, Ltd.

The loss of someone close to us is something that almost all humans will experience, particularly older people, and this can include loss of a partner, a family member or friends. We enter this world as infants biologically preprogrammed to form strong attachments to others, we must therefore also experience the pain of detachment when someone we care for dies. This chapter seeks to explore loss, grief and bereavement in terms of how we understand such concepts as well as the practical issues relevant to nursing care when supporting an older person facing or experiencing loss (Box 29.1).

Society and loss

The past 100 years or so have seen a distinct and noticeable change in the manner that society responds to death and dying in the UK. The relatively recent development of models and theories of how these grief reactions may manifest have influenced the way we view the phenomena of loss, grief and bereavement and suggest how best those affected may be supported (Box 29.2).

Theories of loss, grief and bereavement

Various models have been presented that attempt to describe the complex thoughts and feelings that are experienced when we are bereaved. Elizabeth Kubler Ross is commonly cited as one of the best-known and influential theorists, having developed the five-stage model of grief (Box 29.3) (Kübler Ross, 1969). This model suggests that there are a number of stages experienced by those facing loss, following either the diagnosis of a terminal illness or bereavement. Her model proposed that people experience progressive stages of denial, anger, bargaining, depression and acceptance.

Other 'stage' theories were proposed by John Bowlby and his four stages of grief (Bowlby, 1961) and Colin Murray Parkes' phases of grief theory (Parkes, 1972). Worden (2010) suggested that those experiencing bereavement needed to complete certain 'tasks' in order to 'work through' their grief to find some sense of acceptance and resolution of their loss (Box 29.4).

Stroebe and Schut (1999) developed the 'dual process model'; moving from a perceived linear view of grief, this model suggests that the experience is much more dynamic, with individuals moving between two loss and restoration oriented states (Figure 29.1). Various stimuli (memories, visual reminders, smells, etc.) can act as triggers drawing an individual between one stage or the other. Eventually the bereaved individual will progress to spending more time in the restoration oriented state indicating a positive approach to moving on with one's life.

Other theorists have challenged the long-held notions that grief must be 'worked through' or that stages must be experienced before one feels better, suggesting that traditional theorists have sought to 'pathologise grief'. The absence of a grief reaction can be regarded as 'normal' with individuals who are naturally resilient. Some people do indeed experience very painful and long-lasting grief reactions; however, this is not the norm. Most people 'cope ugly', and perpetuating the notion of having to work through our grief before we feel better can actually be harmful for some individuals.

Factors affecting grief

Five main factors may influence the nature of the grieving process. These include the mode of death, the nature of the attachment, who the person was, historical antecedents, and personality and social variables. Kinghorn and Duncan (2005) also identify a number of elements that may contribute to the process of successfully adjusting to the loss of a loved one (Box 29.5).

These factors may play a part in the process of how individuals adapt to the loss, the length of time this may take and whether individuals experience what may be termed 'complicated grief' (Box 29.6).

Role of the nurse

Most nurses will at some point in their career experience the death of a patient and will be required to support their family and loved ones. They will require the ability to establish and maintain relationships, which in some circumstances will need to be done very quickly. They will need to develop effective interpersonal skills, skills in communicating and giving information as well as the ability to give 'intuitive' support. Nurses need to spend time and be emotionally present with bereaved individuals and allow the bereaved person to set the tone and pace of any interaction or discussion.

Nursing skills when supporting bereaved individuals

- Interpersonal skills.
- Skills in communicating and giving information.
- The ability to give 'intuitive' support.
- Interpersonal skills.
- Skills in communicating and giving information.
- The ability to give 'intuitive' support.
- Caring for the body in a respectful manner.

References

Bowlby, J. (1961) Separation anxiety: a critical review of the literature. *Journal of Child Psychology and Psychiatry* 1(16): 251–269.

Kinghorn, S. and Duncan, F. (2005) Living with loss. In: Lugton, J. and McIntyre, R. (eds) *Palliative Care: the Nurse's Role*, 2nd edn. Edinburgh: Churchill Livingstone, pp. 303–337.

Kübler-Ross, E. (1969) *On Death and Dying*. Routledge

Kübler-Ross, E. (1975) *Death: The Final Stage of Growth*. Englewood Cliffs, NJ: Prentice Hall.

Parkes C.M. (1972) Bereavement: studies in grief in adult life. London: Tavistock.

Stroebe, M. and Schut, H. (1999) The dual process model of coping with bereavement: rationale and description. *Death Studies* 23(3): 197–224.

Worden, J.W. (2010) *Grief Counselling and Grief Therapy*, 4th edn. Hove, East Sussex: Routledge.

30 Safeguarding

Table 30.1 Categories of abuse.

Categories of abuse	Signs and symptoms
Physical: purposeful injury, rough handling; unreasonable or unlawful restraint; forced medication	Bruising; wounds; burns/scalds/welts; restraint marks; visceral injury; fractures, sprains or dislocations; pressure ulcers; overdose; repeat injuries
Emotional/psychological: verbal or psychological abuse; intimidation; threats and other behaviour that affects well-being	Low self-esteem; tearfulness; anger; lack of confidence; social isolation; unmet religious or cultural needs; weight loss or gain and a change in appetite; aches and pains
Financial/material: theft; fraud; misappropriation of funds; exploitation	Missing personal possessions or inexplicable lack of money; rent arrears or unpaid bills; unusual withdrawal of money from bank accounts; mismatch between income and expenditure; missing personal possessions; recent changes in deeds or title to property
Neglect by others/self-neglect: unmet holistic care needs; failure to provide the necessities of life	Dirty torn and worn clothing; poor hygiene; non-attendance for medical appointments; untreated injuries; failure to access care or have equipment to maintain functional independence; malnutrition; accumulation of medicines
Institutional: attitudes and procedures that combine to create an abusive regime	Rough handling; favouritism; regimented routines; no choice; limited range of activity provision; communal use of personal items; breaches of confidentiality; hunger or dehydration; failure to provide adequate privacy and dignity
Sexual: any non-consensual sexual act or behaviour	Incontinence; vaginal or anal bleeding; penile discharge; genital bruising; urinary tract infection; sexually transmitted infection; torn clothing; unusual difficulty in sitting or walking; uncharacteristic use of sexual language or behaviour
Discriminatory: psychological abuse that is racist, sexist or linked to another protected characteristic in the Equality Act 2010	Harassment; slurs and offensive language

Nursing Older People at a Glance, First Edition. Edited by Josie Tetley, Nigel Cox, Kirsten Jack and Gary Witham.
© 2018 John Wiley & Sons, Ltd. Published 2018 by John Wiley & Sons, Ltd.

A life free from abuse is a fundamental human right. All staff working within health services have a responsibility to promote the well-being of those in their care and safeguard them against avoidable harm. Moreover, the Code (Nursing and Midwifery Council, 2015a) reminds nurses to prioritise people and 'make their care and safety your main concern'. Safeguarding older people requires nurses to recognise the vulnerable older person and prevent and respond to harm and abuse (Table 30.1). A nurse's duty of care to patients/service users means upholding their rights in law, treating each individual with dignity and respect, and delivering high-quality care to the best of their ability and speaking out if there are any reasons why they may be unable to do so.

Ageing population

People are living longer, and there are now 11.8 million people (one in six) in the UK who are over 65 years old. Of these, 1.6 million are aged 85 or older. In the next 17 years, the number aged over 65 is projected to rise by more than 40% to just over 16 million (AgeUK, 2017). Not all older people are vulnerable but nurses and others need to be mindful of the needs of those who are or could be, and of the skills and strategies required to keep them safe.

It is important to:
- Recognise potential vulnerability.
- Create a protective environment.

It is essential to:
- Recognise abuse.
- Take appropriate action.

Recognising potential vulnerability and creating a protective environment

People who reside or spend time in health and social care settings may be particularly vulnerable due to their dependency on others for care. They may have frailty, be defenceless, isolated and disabled and worry about being a burden on busy stretched staff. They may have had previously damaging experiences of healthcare and feel unable to raise a concern. They may feel ashamed, worried they will not be believed or may not recognise abuse is taking place. Care staff need to be mindful of power differences, and rough, rushed, impersonal and regimented care has been identified as causing harm (Francis, 2013). In the home setting, people may be vulnerable due to circumstances such as dependency on relatives for care, overcrowding, socioeconomic stress, forced isolation and loneliness.

Nurses can reduce the likelihood of abuse and harm by working with person-centred values that see service users as equal partners in care, and by building strong relationships with family members. Nurses who understand people's needs, culture, likes and dislikes, means and preferred forms of communication limit the risk of harm and strengthen people's resistance and resilience. Isolation increases a person's risk of abuse so nurses can encourage older people to keep active and promote social networking. Good risk assessments should consider what people can do as well as what they cannot do. Nurses need to follow locally agreed policies and procedures and promote a positive culture of care that includes supporting one another as a team, acting as a role model for good practice and cooperating with other professionals to deliver safe and effective care.

Recognising abuse and taking action

Some forms of abuse may be more obvious than others, and it is useful if staff know how an individual normally behaves so they can recognise when something is wrong. Engaging with family and friends is important, and seeing them as part of the 'team' is good practice. Making assumptions is poor practice but where concerns exist doing nothing is never an option. Any action taken to safeguard the older person should meet human rights standards. Staff must act with the consent of the adult with mental capacity, act in the best interests of the person, and for legitimate reasons such as to protect the person or others. Where the person lacks capacity legislation supports decision-making that is in the person's best interests.

Listen to the person's concerns and document accurately, objectively, legibly and contemporaneously. Information must be easily understood by everyone who may read it, including the person at the centre of care, who is legally entitled to request access to their written records. Information must be shared with consent whenever possible, although a person's right to confidentiality may be overridden where sharing is in their best interests. Any judgement of what constitutes best interests will be based on the facts of the case. Seek advice from your local adult safeguarding lead if you are unsure and follow locally agreed policy and procedure. Keep the person safe, and if the person is in immediate danger take action without delay, calling the emergency services if necessary. Remember that staff, including managers, may be perpetrators of abuse and in these instances, staff need to raise and where necessary escalate concerns appropriately within their organisation (Nursing and Midwifery Council, 2015b).

References

AgeUK (2017) Later Life in the United Kingdom. Available at: http://www.ageuk.org.uk/Documents/EN-GB/Factsheets/Later_Life_UK_factsheet.pdf?dtrk=true (accessed 22 September 2017).

Department of Health (2000) No secrets: Guidance on developing and implementing multi-agency policies and procedures to protect vulnerable adults from abuse. London: DoH.

Francis, R. (2013) Report of the Mid Staffordshire NHS Foundation Trust Public Inquiry. London: Stationery Office. Available at: http://webarchive.nationalarchives.gov.uk/20150407084231/http://www.midstaffspublicinquiry.com/report (accessed 6 October 2017).

Nursing and Midwifery Council (2015a) The Code. London: NMC.

Nursing and Midwifery Council (2015b) Raising concerns; Guidance for nurses and midwives. London: NMC.

31 Spiritual beliefs and religious practices

Table 31.1 Key activities for assessing spiritual care.

B	Build a trusting relationship – be prepared to spend time talking with the patient engaging in the use of effective communication skills
R	Respect, respond and react appropriately to differences in thought and ideas about spiritual/religious matters
A	Actively listen to patients. Ask appropriate questions to deepen understanding and develop a plan of action to meet their spirituality/religious needs
V	Value and validate the individuality of the patient's need to express their spirituality/religious practices. Ensure that privacy, time and environment are accessible and enable fulfilment of need
E	Empower and encourage patient involvement in formulating a plan of action. Collaboratively evaluate the effectiveness of the plan

Nursing Older People at a Glance, First Edition. Edited by Josie Tetley, Nigel Cox, Kirsten Jack and Gary Witham.
© 2018 John Wiley & Sons, Ltd. Published 2018 by John Wiley & Sons, Ltd.

Considering the spiritual and religious needs of older people can positively influence their capacity for coping with ill health and disability. However, the ways in which nurses might meet these needs in healthcare settings are less well understood. For example, a survey of 4000 nurses confirmed that meeting such needs improves the overall quality of the patient's experience of care. However, only 5% of the respondents felt that this goal was achievable within healthcare settings (Funning, 2010).

Due to the subjective nature of spirituality and religion, it might be difficult to provide formal education and practical guidance to healthcare professionals on how to ensure patients' needs are met. Lack of formal education might contribute to discomfort when nurses are assessing and providing spiritual and religious care. In anticipating such needs, one has to acknowledge that, although religious practices and spiritual beliefs are often linked, they are not necessarily synonymous.

Of the two terms 'religion' is much easier to define, being associated with a belief in a supernatural power. However, although religions are sometimes symbolised by engaging in routines and ritualistic practices, it would be a mistake to assume adherence to these practices is based solely on religious affiliation. Spirituality is a complex term, encompassing a wider remit but is linked to the consideration, meaning and purpose of life. For many patients this could focus on their personal and moral values for living, interconnections with family/significant others/the divine, careers, achievements in life, passion for creativity and aesthetic aspects of life (Sartori, 2010).

Nurses might avoid undertaking spiritual/religious assessment and perceive that to be the duty of a trained clergy person (Barlow, 2015). Practical guidance for the undertaking of such assessment is considered below. Koenig (2007) suggests that assessment should be:

- brief;
- person-centred;
- easy to remember;
- able to elicit appropriate information.

There are helpful tools devised to support the assessment of spiritual and religious issues, for example 'HOPE' (Anandarajah and Hight, 2001). Utilisation of such assessment tools can support health professionals in asking focused questions, whilst gaining insight into the important aspects of spiritual and religious matters, needed to devise appropriate plans for intervention. For example, using the 'HOPE' tool (Anandarajah and Hight, 2001), the practitioner could focus conversations on the following aspects:

H – Sources of hope, strength, comfort, meaning, peace, love and connection.

O – The role and the significance of organised religion for the patient.

P – Personal spirituality and/or religious practices that the patient engages in.

E – Effects and influence that such beliefs may have on medical care and end of life decisions.

Such conversations can provide opportunities for the patient to share their views, discuss their needs and to plan meaningful intervention in respect of spirituality and religious matters. It is the responsibility of the health professional to create an environment conducive for this to happen (Barlow, 2015).

Fundamental activities that will assist health professionals in engaging patients in talking about spiritual and religious matters can be memorised by using the mnemonic 'BRAVE', summarised in Table 31.1. Taking a 'BRAVE' approach the health professional should be committed to:

B – Building a trusting relationship. Must spend time talking with the patient, engaging in the use of effective communication skills. The use of open-ended questions, reflecting and paraphrasing conversation content will ensure that the patient is fully understood, enhancing your ability to intervene appropriately.

R – Respecting and responding appropriately to differences in thoughts and ideas about spiritual/religious matters; especially those ideas that may challenge our own beliefs. Remembering that the goal is to accept and acknowledge the patient's stance and discuss practical ways in which adherence to such beliefs can be made possible within care settings.

A – Actively listening to patients, asking appropriate questions to deepen understanding. Active listening is more than hearing; it calls for the professional to:

- give undivided attention;
- show that you are listening;
- provide feedback;
- defer judgement;
- respond appropriately.

V – Valuing the individuality and autonomy of the patients to express their spirituality/religious practices. Ensuring that privacy, time and the environment are accessible and enable fulfilment of need. Include meaningful others in the process with the patient's consent.

E – Empowering and encouraging the individual's involvement in formulating a current plan of action. Ensuring if the context demands, that end of life wishes/plans are openly discussed with the patient and meaningful others. Collaboratively, evaluating the effectiveness of the plan of intervention in meeting the unique spiritual/religious needs of the patient.

In addition to the aforementioned activities, when assessing spiritual/religious needs of the older person, it is vital to appreciate and accommodate the potential impact of cognitive/physical impairment, and where necessary adapt the assessment accordingly.

In conclusion, when addressing the spiritual/religious needs of patients, it is necessary to recognise that this aspect of care is not prescriptive and only becomes meaningful if the individuality of expression is proactively encouraged, appreciated and supported by healthcare professionals and carers. Ultimately, planning and engagement in providing good spiritual care has the desired effect of enhancing patients' ability to cope with illness, as well as enhancing the experience of care.

References

Anandarajah, G. and Hight, E. (2001) Spirituality and medical practice: the HOPE questions as a practical tool for spiritual assessment. *American Family Physician* 63: 81–89.

Barlow, A. (2015) Spirituality in nursing. Allnurses. Available at: http://allnurses.com/nursing-and-spirituality/spirituality-in-nursing-646693.html (accessed 4 October 2017).

Funning, B. (2010) Spirituality. *RCN Bulletin* 19 May, p. 5.

Koenig, H.G (2007) *Spirituality in Patient Care: How, When Where and What?* Philadelphia: Templeton Fountain Press.

Sartori, P. (2010) Spirituality 1: Should spiritual and religious beliefs be part of patient care? *Nursing Times* 106(28): 14–17.

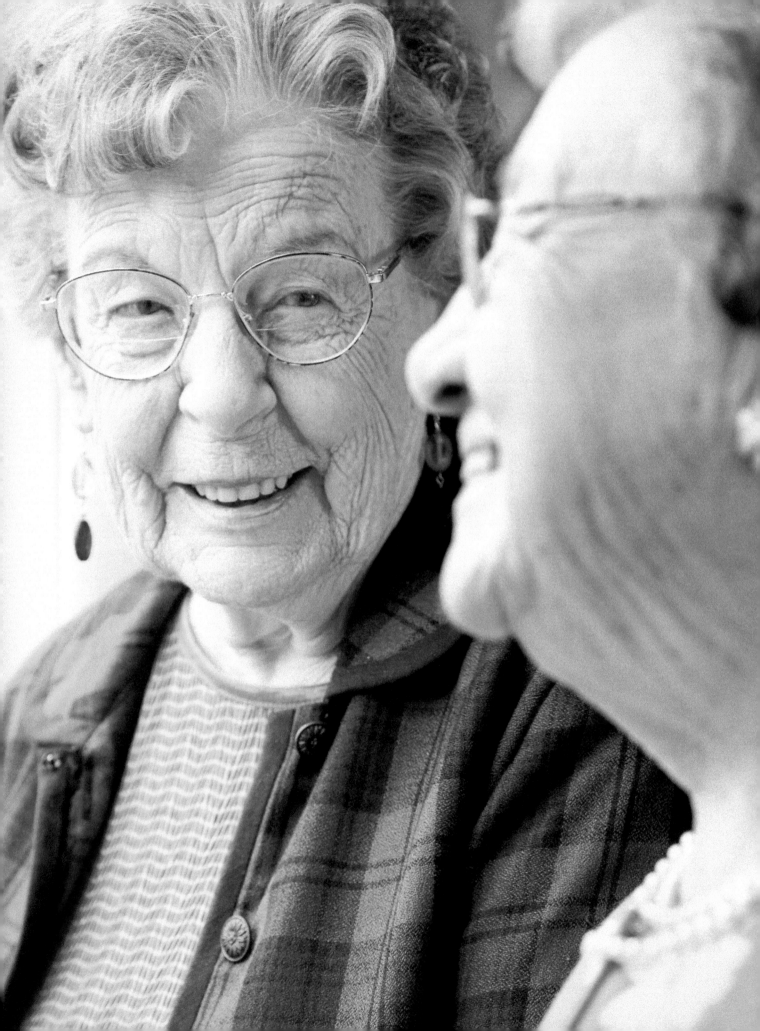

Equality and diversity in practice

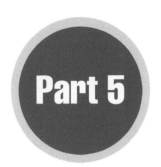

Part 5

Chapters

Promoting dignified care for diverse communities

Figure 32.1 An outline of how to adopt a positive interaction to make cultural delivery of care effective. Source: Adapted from Kitwood (1997).

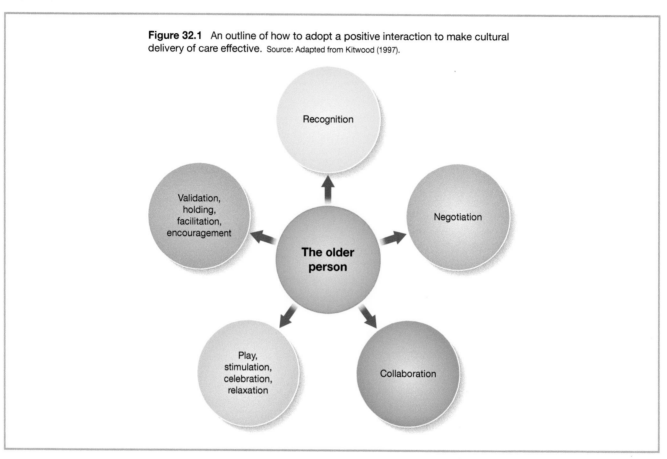

Culturally sensitive care is characterised by a person-centred, flexible, respectful and client-empowering attitude (Tucker *et al.*, 2011). Effective, culturally sensitive health professionals would be those who adopt an attitude that allows them to want to understand, appreciate and work with individuals from cultures other than their own. It is more than understanding dietary restrictions or modesty dress codes that need to be followed. It is an attitude facilitated by a team approach of being aware and accepting of cultural differences, self-awareness and a desire to get to know a patient's culture and creative adaptation of skills to individuals.

When giving consideration to the diverse needs within any population, it becomes a limiting exercise only to consider obvious or ethnic differences as a marker for assessing cultural difference. There is also a need to take into account cultural diversity within the majority population. This would include varying life experiences such as differences in geography (e.g. individuals who have lived in remote rural areas), sexuality (e.g. LGBT communities), religious or spiritual beliefs, and socioeconomic background amongst others. Even within these groups there are wide variations in cultural practice, and the fundamental requirement in providing culturally sensitive care to the older person is to provide person-centred care (Zimmerman *et al.*, 2005).

In terms of ethnic or religious differences, there are many websites, books and guidelines that you can refer to in order to gain an understanding of an individual's acknowledged identity. It is important to note, however, that almost all cultural and religious practices are socially variable depending on the geography, history and lifestyle of the community from which that individual person originates. This is exemplified by the variety of ways in which religions such as Christianity or Islam are practised around the UK, never mind the world. Also, lack of a religious belief does not exclude a person from having spiritual convictions that affect the way that person has chosen to lead their life.

Figure 32.1, an adaptation of Kitwood's (1997, p. 15) seminal work on person-centredness, provides a general outline in how to adopt a positive interaction to make cultural delivery of care effective.

Recognition: Acknowledge the individual by their preferred name/title (in some cultures, older people, even if unrelated, may be referred to as Uncle, Aunty, Grandma, and so forth. Make it known to all staff/be aware of non-aggressive eye contact/acknowledge presence even if not interacting directly.

Negotiation: Ask for preferences, choices and needs even when there is a lack of common language or cognitive impairment. Try to negotiate with carers or significant others regarding preferences.

Collaboration: Working with third sector or voluntary organisations may further promote person-centred cultural care and support collaboration with family or carers.

Play, stimulation, celebration, relaxation: Engage in activities and interactions that are meaningful to the individual and stimulate their senses (e.g. music, festivals: ensure these are correct to the person involved, do not assume).

Validation, holding, facilitation, encouragement: Try to be empathetic and affirm the person's preferred identity (e.g. preferred sexual characteristics for a person who is transgender). Try to acknowledge a patient's expressions of emotion, which may differ from your own, and provide physical contact beyond essential care. Providing a safe place for the person to express themselves is important. People may be gently persuaded to engage in activities that are culturally acceptable, but the nurse needs to be mindful that some activities may never have been acceptable to the person (e.g. dancing or singing with people of the opposite sex).

Asking the person or their significant caregiver (if required) will improve your understanding of that person's preference or perspective rather than just assuming that a set of written guidelines or popularly expressed beliefs applies to all. However, an individual's cultural identity is a complex multi-layered issue, sometimes obvious but mainly subtle and unconscious. It will have changed, modified and adapted over time by being influenced externally through history, politics and through the power of media (Triandis and Trafimow, 2001). The result of memory loss and some adoption of older cultural practices can result in challenges and distress for family and health professionals.

An understanding of personal history is of particular importance for professional carers, as it will be a starting point for planning culturally sensitive person-centred care. For example, the historical understanding of the present-day elderly population within the Orthodox Jewish population would be to acknowledge that some of the elderly individuals who have dementia from this community may have been survivors of the Holocaust in Nazi Germany. People from all communities may have had traumatic experiences as children, and this knowledge will help with planning a more sensitive and gentle approach to care.

In summary, providing effective culturally sensitive care requires a team approach of genuine interest and empathy to comprehend those internal and external dimensions by which the older person understands themselves and others around them.

References

Kitwood, T. (1997) *Dementia Reconsidered: The Person Comes First.* Buckingham: Open University Press.

Triandis, H.C. and Trafimow, D. (2001) Culture and its implications for intergroup behaviour. In: Brown, R. and GaertnerS.L. (eds) *Blackwell Handbook of Social Psychology: Intergroup Processes.* Oxford: Blackwell Publishers, pp. 367–385.

Tucker, C.M., Marsiske, M., Rice, K.G., Jones, J.D. and Herman, K.C. (2011) Patient-centered culturally sensitive health care: model testing and refinement. *Health Psychology* 30: 342–350.

Zimmerman, S., Williams, C.S., Reed, P.S., Boustani, M., Preisser, J.S., Heck, E. and Sloane, P.D. (2005) Attitudes, stress, and satisfaction of staff who care for residents with dementia. *The Gerontologist* 45 (Suppl. 1): 96–105.

Supporting good mental health in older people

Figure 33.1 Model for mental health and mental illness. Source: Enns (2016). Reproduced with permission of Elsevier.

Optimal mental health 'flourishing'

A person who has a diagnosable mental illness, but has high levels of mental well-being (e.g. sense of purpose, participation in society, positive self-concept)

A person who has a high level of mental well-being (e.g. positive self-concept, relationships with others, sense of purpose) and no mental illness

Severe mental illness

No mental illness

A person who has a diagnosable mental illness, and has low levels of mental well-being (e.g. low self-esteem, inability to perform important life roles)

A person who has no diagnosable mental illness, but has low levels of mental well-being (e.g. feelings of emptiness, stagnation, social isolation)

Minimal mental health 'languishing'

Key points

Five ways of maintaining mental well-being can be summarised as follows:
1. **Connect** (e.g. joining a group or interest group).
2. **Keep learning** (e.g. a new hobby).
3. **Be active** (e.g. walking, moving more).
4. **Give to others** (e.g. support and conversation with friends and family).
5. **Take notice** (do activities that remove you from the day-to-day stresses of life).

In terms of mental health, depression, panic disorder and social phobia are the most common challenges affecting functioning and quality of life in older life, particularly in the presence of frailty. Mental health can be viewed as a spectrum and independent of any underlying mental condition. Keyes (2002) has developed the dual continuum model of mental health. Within this model mental health and mental illness are conceptualised as two distinct dimensions characterised by both affect and functioning in life (Figure 33.1). Therefore being mentally healthy (*flourishing*) is distinguished as a state where people combine a high level of subjective well-being with optimal levels of psychological and social functioning (Key points), and *languishing* refers to a state where these constructs are at low levels. Mental illness is related to mental health but individuals who exhibit symptoms of mental illness may also be highly functional, and conversely, people without mental illness can be languishing.

Depression

In terms of supporting older people with depression, longer interventions (more than 3 months) have a more positive effect involving meaningful social activities. These should be tailored to meet the older person's individual abilities and needs (Forsman *et al.*, 2011). Educational interventions have also proved to be effective in mental health promotion through a reduction in loneliness and social isolation amongst older people. Indeed, social support is a protective factor against depression and helps maintain good mental health in older age. Interventions that have been used to prevent depression are:

- Physical activity.
- Cognitive behavioural therapy (CBT).
- Other educational approaches.
- Reminiscence – a type of story-telling that recounts past personal experiences and events.
- Life review – a more structured, systematic intervention.

There is clear evidence that a structured intervention to promote physical activity (that takes account of ability) can reduce the severity of depression in older people (Netz *et al.*, 2005). It is suggested that two sessions a week for 45 minutes duration is the minimum level to affect mental health. Cognitive behavioural therapy and educational interventions that reframe situations can reduce negative thinking especially if this is associated with multiple losses from chronic disease/disability. Reminiscence has been shown to have a moderate influence on life satisfaction and emotional well-being (particularly in community-dwelling adults rather than in adults living in nursing or residential care), although life review had greater significance for psychological well-being than simple reminiscence.

Structured life review is an intervention that is implemented on an individual basis with the reviewer and listener. Participants reflect on the key aspects of the reviewer's life in an evaluative and supportive way. Through gentle probing and questioning the listener assesses physical, psychological and cognitive functioning. This process is structured to about six to eight 1-hour sessions starting with childhood, family and home to adulthood and finally a summary and evaluation of this process. The Life Review and Experiencing Form can be used as a guide (see Haight, 2007) and other props like music or pictures can be utilised.

Anxiety and associated disorders

Anxiety disorders have been shown to reduce well-being, health-related quality of life and increase health utilisation and disability in older age. The evidence for effective interventions to manage anxiety is similar to that for treating depression, with cognitive behavioural therapy, antidepressant drug therapy and exercise reducing anxiety in older people. In terms of behavioural techniques, relaxation therapy seems to be the most effective component of CBT for those in later life. There is also evidence to suggest that mindfulness can be an effective technique for anxiety reduction. Mindfulness meditation supports a focused, non-judgemental awareness of present moment experiences as a way to counter worry and anxiety generated from future concerns.

Mindfulness-based stress reduction (MBSR)

A systematic, group-based intervention that introduces the concept of mindfulness and nurtures its development through regular practice of techniques such as yoga, mindful breathing and various types of meditation. Mindfulness meditation has been used within diverse populations and with older people with a wide array of medical conditions. As a method to ground our thoughts, emotions and sensations it can be adapted and applied regardless of any underlying physical needs. Similarly, the attitudes cultivated in mindfulness meditation such as acceptance, patience and compassion are not linked to a particular population or group and therefore have more universal cultural transference.

References

Enns, J., Holmqvist, M., Wener, P., Halas, G., Rothney, J., Schultz, A. et al. (2016) Mapping interventions that promote mental health in the general population: a scoping review of reviews. *Preventive Medicine* 87: 70–80.

Forsman, A.F., Nordmyr, J. and Wahlbeck, K. (2011) Psychosocial interventions for the promotion of mental health and the prevention of depression among older adults. *Health Promotion International* 26(S1): i85–i107

Haight, B.K. (2007) *Transformational Reminiscence: Life Story Work*. New York: Springer Publishing Co.

Keyes, C.L. (2002) The mental health continuum: from languishing to flourishing in life. *Journal of Health and Social Behaviour* 43(2:, 207–222.

Netz, Y., Wu, M-J., Becker, B.J. and Tenenbaum, G. (2005) Physical activity and psychological well-being in advanced age: a meta-analysis of intervention studies. *Psychology and Aging* 20(2): 272–284.

Further resources

BeMindful website (http://bemindful.co.uk/).

The Free Mindfulness Project (http://www.freemindfulness.org/download).

Mindfulness

Means paying attention in a particular way, on purpose, in the present moment, non-judgmentally.

Source: Jon Kabat-Zinn

34 Ageing without children

Box 34.1 Diversity and difference in forms of parenthood. Source: Adapted from Marchbank and Letherby (2007).

- Biological parent(s) who raise their children.
- Biological parent(s) who do not raise their children (e.g. gamete donors).
- Biological parents who have fractured relationships with their children (e.g. through divorce).
- People who believe they are biological parents but are not: e.g. a man whose partner was impregnated by another man.
- People who adopt or foster.
- Social or step-parent with no biological children of his or her own.
- Lesbian or gay people who may co-parent a partner's biological child.
- Parents of a surrogate child.

Box 34.2 Older people without children and family.

Voluntarily childless: People who decided they did not want children. There is a vast range of reasons why a person may decide not to have children, from their own poor experience of parenting to concerns about the size of the global population. Terms associated with voluntary childlessness include chosen-childless and childfree.

Involuntarily childless: People who wanted to become parents but for a variety of reasons did not. These range from unsuccessful infertility treatment to economic reasons. For example, a person may have had to delay starting a family because they had to move to find employment. Terms associated with involuntary childlessness include childless-by-circumstance and childless.

Childless parent: People who are parents but, for a variety of reasons, have no contact with their children. For example, their child may have died or their child lives far away. Parental separation often means that the biological father or social father loses or has no contact with their children.

Estranged parent: People who are parents but who do not have contact with their adult children. There are many reasons why people are not in contact with their adult children, for example, through family dispute.

Singleton child: A person who was the only child may have few or no distant relatives.

Bereavement: A person whose partner has died may lose contact with their partner's family. This is especially important if the surviving person has no family or close friends. Older men tend to have smaller social networks than women.

Over the last few decades there has been a change in the shape of families, one that can be linked to a long-term decline in fertility rate, the rise in the age of mortality, economics, and increases in divorce rates and stepfamilies (Box 34.1). Not only are families smaller than previously, but also there is an increase in the number of people ageing without children. By 2030 it is estimated there will be over a million people in the UK aged 65 or over who are childless (McNeil and Hunter, 2014). The childless are a much under-researched group and as a result they are often absent from both policy and practice information, and this has implications for nursing practice when caring for this group. Research shows that older childless people are not disadvantaged when they are well but should they need help they are more quickly taken into formal care settings than people with family (Albertini and Mencarini, 2014). Moreover, as men tend have smaller social networks and are more likely to be estranged from adult children than women, they are more likely to be placed in residential care than their female equivalents (Arber *et al.*, 2003).

Who is childless?

Childlessness is found in every society, and reactions from others vary from hostility to sympathy. Childlessness is mostly associated with those who do not have biological children because they either 'chose' to be childless or are 'involuntarily' childless. There are many reasons why people may choose not to have children. It might be due to a poor experience in their upbringing, a fear of childbirth, or that becoming a parent just didn't feel right. There are many influences on why a person who wanted or expected to be a parent does not become one. For example, older LGBTQ+ people have little choice about whether they have children because of cultural and social discrimination. Other circumstances that may impact on a person's childlessness include economics, relationship issues and bereavement (Box 34.2).

What do older childless people want?

A survey conducted by the charity Ageing Without Children (2016) found that childless people reported a number of issues, which have implications for healthcare professionals.

Firstly, at times childless people felt invisible, and often health and care services generally assume that all older people have adult children and/or grandchildren. Many reports on ageing do not mention the childless but focus on adult children as the main source of support and care. Secondly, the language used in everyday conversation and in official documents can be hurtful to childless older people. Older people are often referred to as 'granny' or 'grandad' and this may feel inappropriate and isolating to those without children. Childless older people are as diverse a group as any other, and insensitive or unthoughtful comments reinforce discrimination and exclusion. Thirdly, because they were childless many people in this group were seen as being available to care for ageing parents. Consequently, many reported anxiety regarding who would care for them and be an advocate for their wishes and views. This was connected to a deep fear of dementia. Older childless people worry about how they are going to manage practical issues as they age and how they can access services. Here the provision of memory boxes and of a record of personal preferences through management folders may be of some help.

Older childless people have multiple concerns related to ageing and how they will be treated should they become physically or mentally unwell. It is important that nurses do not assume that all older people have families who can be called upon when needed. The need to treat others as unique individuals is paramount to avoid stereotyping and the making of assumptions relating to older people having children. Nurses need to remain self-aware and never assume that all older people have children or are grandparents. Older childless people have the same issues as any other older person. It is important to appreciate that older childless people have the added concerns of being invisible to policy makers and service providers and, through discrimination, exclusion and isolation, might feel like 'outsiders' in the social world.

References

Ageing without Children (2016) *Our Voices*. London: AWOC. Available at: https://awoc.org/our-voices-2/ (accessed 2 October 2017).

Albertini, M. and Mencarini, L. (2014) Childlessness and support networks in later life: new pressures on familistic welfare states? *Journal of Family Issues* 35: 331–357.

Arber, S., Davidson, K. and Ginn, J. (2003) Changing approaches to gender and later life. In: Arber, S., Davidson, K. and Ginn, J. (eds), *Gender and Ageing. Changing Roles and Relationships*. Maidenhead: Open University Press, pp. 1–14.

Marchbank, J. and Letherby, G. (2007) *Introduction to Gender: Social Science Perspectives*. Pearson Education.

McNeil, C. and Hunter, J. (2014) The Generation Strain. The collective solutions to care in an ageing society. London: Institute for Public Policy Research.

35 Lesbian, gay, bisexual and transgendered older people

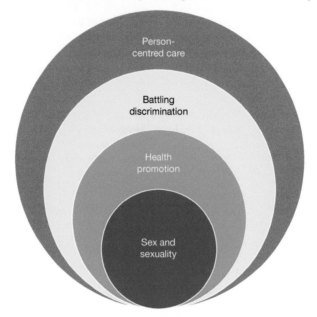

Figure 35.1 Important factors when assessing and delivering care to older individuals who identify as being from the LGBT community.

Person-centred care

Battling discrimination

Health promotion

Sex and sexuality

Nursing Older People at a Glance, First Edition. Edited by Josie Tetley, Nigel Cox, Kirsten Jack and Gary Witham.
© 2018 John Wiley & Sons, Ltd. Published 2018 by John Wiley & Sons, Ltd.

Person-centred care

While attitudes towards the lesbian, gay, bisexual and transgendered (LGBT) community are changing in a positive way, some older members of the community have lived with oppression for many years of their life and this leads to reluctance to disclose personal details to healthcare professionals and carers. Discrimination in the LGBT community can have far-reaching effects, ultimately impacting on the health of the individual. The consequences of even the mildest form of discrimination can result in depression and a deterioration in the physical health of the individual, making an anti-discriminatory person-centred approach essential when focusing upon the health of an individual who identifies themselves as part of the LGBT community. Changes in law and social acceptance over the past 50 years have meant there is an increasing number of the population who are happy to identify as LGBT, yet are not provided with the appropriate care to fulfil their needs. A person-centred approach needs to be implemented to ensure that the individuals' needs are met in the delivery of their health requirements (Figure 35.1). Hughes and Cartwright (2014) highlight that LGBT individuals are sometimes unaware of issues such as legal rights around end of life care, and issues such as these should be raised by healthcare practitioners to ensure that planning options are explored. While those receiving care are encouraged to express their religious and spiritual beliefs, the same cannot be said for their sexuality or alternative gender. Stonewall emphasise that half of all people aged over 55 who identify as LGB feel that their sexual orientation would impact negatively on them as they became older (Guasp, 2013).

Battling discrimination

To enable those who deliver healthcare to older LGBT individuals it is important first to understand the health needs of those individuals; this relies upon health education and a knowledge base. Cornelius and Carrick (2015) identify that currently in healthcare there is a lack of knowledge and sensitivity around this topic, which can lead to health disparities. Failing to address someone's sexuality and their sexual needs is a failure to deliver person-centred care. People express their sexuality in differing ways, so it is important to have a non-judgemental approach to the ways in which individuals identify with their sexuality. This relies on self-awareness during all interactions. However a person identifies themselves, the care they receive must be tailored to their needs with care and compassion, and stereotyping should be avoided at all times (Carabez et al., 2015).

To help educate and understand the different terminologies around the LGBT community, and sexuality in general, it is helpful for nurses to recognise terms so they can better deliver person-centred care, and have an open dialogue with their patient showing an understanding.

Health promotion/sex and sexuality

Older people can be sexually active into their 90s and encouraging these relationships is beneficial to promote mental health and well-being. Nurses should encourage discussion around sexual needs in order to identify risky behaviours and promote prevention techniques. With 28% of all men who have sex with men (MSM) living with a diagnosed HIV infection in the UK being over 50 years of age (Public Health England, 2014), there is a necessity to actively promote the sexual health of the older individual. Many charities offer support for the LGBT community with specific health needs and issues, and referral to these can be made easily by nurses.

The key to treating the LGBT older person according to their individual needs is to ensure that we are treating them equitably as opposed to equally. Equitable treatment of the individual means that we fairly and impartially address their requirements, not ignoring their sexuality, but embracing it and addressing it. The only way of encompassing all factors in caring for the LGBT person is to communicate effectively with them and be open to talking about their sexuality, lifestyle, background and future needs. This would normally be performed as part of a nursing assessment, and while this kind of questioning may not be part of any standard assessment, nurses must use their initiative to assess beyond a tick box exercise. Connolly and Lynch (2016) highlight that some in the LGBT community fear coming out to healthcare professionals due to judgement or the possibility of being open to excessive investigations. To overcome a potential fear such as this it will be necessary to explain fully to patients exactly why knowing if they are LGBT is relevant to the care being delivered.

Conclusions

It is crucial to adopt an open approach when caring for older people who identify themselves as LGBT. Having an understanding of the differing terminology that the individual may use to identify themselves or their sexuality can be helpful and aid effective communication. A collaborative approach can support person-centred care, and the nurse can liaise with local charities and support groups that offer specific help for the LGBT community's health needs.

References

Carabez, R., Pellegrini, M., Mankovitz, A., Eliason, M., Ciano, M. and Scott, M. (2015) "Never in all my years…": Nurses' education about LGBT health. *Journal of Professional Nursing* 31(4): 323–329.

Connolly, M.P. and Lynch, K. (2016) Is being gay bad for your health and wellbeing? Cultural issues affecting gay men accessing and using health services in the Republic of Ireland. *Journal of Research in Nursing* 21(3): 177–196.

Cornelius, J.B. and Carrick, J. (2015) A survey of nursing students' knowledge of and attitudes toward LGBT health care concerns. *Nursing Education Perspectives* May/June, pp. 176–178.

Guasp, A. (2013) Gay and Bisexual Men's Health Survey. Stonewall. Available at: http://www.stonewall.org.uk/sites/default/files/Gay_and_Bisexual_Men_s_Health_Survey__2013_.pdf (accessed 25 September 2017).

Hughes, M. and Cartwright, C. (2014) LGBT people's knowledge of and preparedness to discuss end-of-life care planning options. *Health and Social Care in the Community* 22(5): 545–552.

Public Health England (2014) Promoting the health and wellbeing of gay, bisexual and other men who have sex with men. London: PHE.

36 Older people with learning disabilities

Box 36.1 The Mental Capacity Act five key principles. Source: Department of Health (2005). Contains public sector information licensed under the Open Government Licence v3.0.

Principle 1: A presumption of capacity – every adult has the right to make their own decision and society must assume that the person has the capacity to make that decision. One cannot, for example, make an automatic assumption that a person is unable to make a decision because of a learning disability.

Principle 2: Support for decisions – every possible means of supporting a person to reach a decision must be used. Even if some degree of lack of capacity is established one must still involve the person in the decision as far as is practicably possible.

Principle 3: Support for the right to make unwise decisions – people may make decisions that are considered by others as unwise. This should not be automatically assumed to prove lack of capacity.

Principle 4: Best interests of the person – every action or intervention taken on behalf of the person must be in their best interests.

Principle 5: Less restrictive option – any action or intervention should interfere with a person's freedom to act and their rights as little as possible.

Box 36.2 Putting it all into action.

What is the weight of the decision being made?

- Everyone is capable of making some decisions (e.g. the decision to roll over in bed to change position). Some people may find it more challenging to reach a decision on a more complex matter (e.g. Do I take the train to work or drive in, which is quicker, and risk being late as I might not be able to find a parking space?).

What is the context of the decision?

- How can we best facilitate communication about this issue?
- How can we find out about the person's thoughts – this will include consideration of their values and beliefs, hopes and aspirations.
- What are the likely impacts on the person once the decision is reached?

What documentation is required?

- How is assessment conducted, who was involved?
- Documents clearly show the outcome of the discussions.
- The person's file contains accurate, contemporaneous records of the decision-making process.

Who needs to be involved in the discussion process?

- Key family members.
- Advocate.
- Health and social care staff.
- Other professionals.

In terms of definition, 'learning disability' means a combination of impaired intelligence and social functioning that started in childhood (Department of Health, 2001). It is important to understand that people with learning disabilities are a diverse group of people from all sections of society, that the population profile is changing, and diagnosis, if desirable at all, is not always straightforward.

The numbers of people with learning disabilities are increasing in western society (Kelly *et al.*, 2007). This increase is partly because populations are growing as people live longer, but also because people with complex health conditions and disabilities in childhood are much more likely to survive into adulthood than was previously the case. People with learning disabilities share many of the same issues experienced by other people as they get older but there are some areas that are notably different for them as a group. Heller *et al.* (2014) discuss three main areas of importance to age and learning disability: people with learning disabilities tend to age earlier; they tend to have more health problems; and they have different family patterns than the general population.

People with learning disabilities tend to age earlier than other people

There are a number of reasons why people with learning disabilities are more likely to age earlier than other people. There is evidence to suggest that people with certain syndromes are more likely to develop dementia much earlier than others and that people with Down syndrome are particularly at risk from developing dementia (Visser *et al.*, 1997). There are also a range of health factors that affect people with learning disabilities that mean that some may age earlier than others. People with learning disabilities may live lives associated with poverty and are affected by the same factors that link poverty and ageing as others in society (Northway, 2001).

People with learning disabilities tend to have more health problems than other people

This poor health status is due to a combination of unhealthy lifestyles (exacerbated by limited access to paid and meaningful employment), poor access to health services, and a range of physical conditions related to specific disabilities. The result of this is that people with learning disabilities develop into their later years from a position of vulnerability rather than strength.

People with learning disabilities tend to have different family patterns than other people

The fact that people with learning disabilities are likely to have different family patterns than others is a most striking difference from the general population. While it is important to understand that there are exceptions it is more likely that people with learning disabilities continue to live with their parents well into adult-

hood, and sometimes into old age. A possible consequence of this situation is that services may not be aware of people with a learning disability in their area until such times as the parents can no longer manage, or they pass away and services become involved in an emergency.

Implications

It is important to be guided by the principle that the main similarity between people with learning disabilities and other people is that they need to be treated as individuals (Box 36.1). In order to ensure that older people with a learning disability are supported and enabled to retain maximum autonomy, and remain as participants in their communities, then healthcare services must address the following:

• First, healthcare monitoring processes and interventions must be predicated on a recognition that people with a learning disability have a range of health issues requiring action.
• Second, healthcare interventions must be based upon a proactive approach that incorporates meaningful assessment beginning in early adulthood and has long-term planning as its central precept (Box 36.2).

Conclusions

People with learning disabilities are a diverse group of people from all sections of society who tend to age earlier than other people. They have more health problems than other people and often have more than one health issue affecting them at the same time. People with learning disabilities are more likely to live with their parents until well into middle age, or with groups of people of a similar age, and are less likely to be married than other people.

References

Department of Health (2001) Valuing People: A New Strategy for Learning Disability for the 21st Century. London: Department of Health.

Department of Health (2005). Mental Capacity Act. London: Department of Health.

Heller, T., Fisher, D., Marks, B. and Hsieh, K. (2014) Interventions to promote health: Crossing networks of intellectual and developmental disabilities and aging. *Disability and Health Journal* 7(1) (Suppl.): S24–S32.

Kelly, F., Kelly, C. and Craig, S. (2007) Annual Report of the National Intellectual Disability Database Committee 2007 (no. 2009 034X). Dublin: Health Research Board.

Northway, R. (2001) Poverty as a practice issue for learning disability nurses. *British Journal of Nursing* 10(18): 1188–1192.

Visser, F.E., Aldenkamp, A.P., Van Huffelen, A.C., et al. (1997) Prospective study of the prevalence of Alzheimer-type dementia in institutionalized individuals with Down syndrome. *American Journal on Mental Retardation* 101: 400–412.

37 Substance misuse (drugs and alcohol)

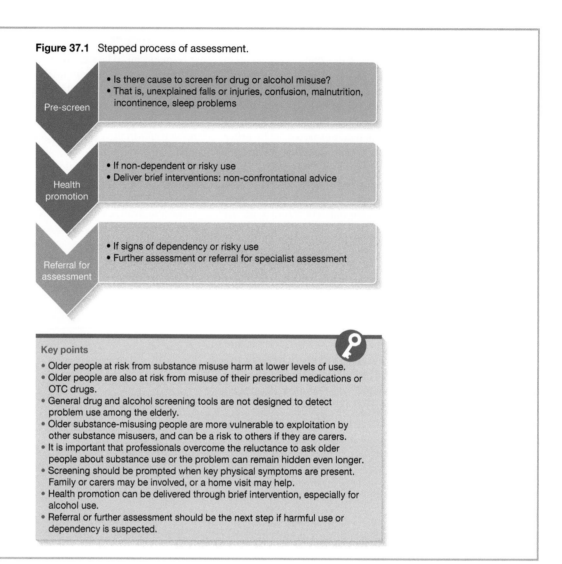

Figure 37.1 Stepped process of assessment.

Pre-screen
- Is there cause to screen for drug or alcohol misuse?
- That is, unexplained falls or injuries, confusion, malnutrition, incontinence, sleep problems

Health promotion
- If non-dependent or risky use
- Deliver brief interventions: non-confrontational advice

Referral for assessment
- If signs of dependency or risky use
- Further assessment or referral for specialist assessment

Key points
- Older people at risk from substance misuse harm at lower levels of use.
- Older people are also at risk from misuse of their prescribed medications or OTC drugs.
- General drug and alcohol screening tools are not designed to detect problem use among the elderly.
- Older substance-misusing people are more vulnerable to exploitation by other substance misusers, and can be a risk to others if they are carers.
- It is important that professionals overcome the reluctance to ask older people about substance use or the problem can remain hidden even longer.
- Screening should be prompted when key physical symptoms are present. Family or carers may be involved, or a home visit may help.
- Health promotion can be delivered through brief intervention, especially for alcohol use.
- Referral or further assessment should be the next step if harmful use or dependency is suspected.

Isn't substance misuse a problem for everybody? What's special about older people?

Older people who misuse substances have more unmet needs than younger people. They have been a marginalised population for service provision and research evidence for a long time (Ayres *et al.*, 2012). Health advice, screening tools, risk indicators and treatment approaches for substance misuse are more likely to be targeted at younger people (Wadd *et al.*, 2011). Deaths related to substance use are higher among older people compared to younger people (Royal College of Psychiatrists, 2011). While the number of young people starting to use heroin and crack cocaine is declining, most people in substance misuse treatment are now over 40 (Public Health England, 2013). Older people who

misuse substances are less healthy than younger people and more vulnerable to other health problems.

What do we mean by 'substance misuse' in older populations?

We usually think of 'substance misuse' as addiction to street or recreational drugs like heroin, cocaine or cannabis. We might also include alcohol dependency and binge drinking as 'misuse'. However, among the older age groups we can include misuse of prescription medications and non-dependent harmful alcohol use as well (see Key points box) (National Treatment Agency, 2011). Also, remember that many grandparents have care of children. In these cases, older age substance misuse is also an issue for safeguarding if the older person is intoxicated while supervising young grandchildren.

Nursing Older People at a Glance, First Edition. Edited by Josie Tetley, Nigel Cox, Kirsten Jack and Gary Witham.
© 2018 John Wiley & Sons, Ltd. Published 2018 by John Wiley & Sons, Ltd.

How are older people at risk from substance misuse?

Substance-related physical disease, such as coronary heart disease, liver disease, cancer of the bowel and oesophagus, and alcohol-related dementia, is more prevalent in older people.

> Because of physiological changes associated with ageing, older people are at increased risk of adverse physical effects of substance misuse, even at relatively modest levels of intake
>
> *Royal College of Psychiatrists, 2011, p. 7*

- Blood alcohol concentration is higher in older people than younger people for the same amount consumed. So, recommended 'safe' limits may be too high for older people.
- The blood–brain barrier is less effective at protecting the brain from the toxins in drugs and alcohol so there is greater vulnerability to confusion.
- Older people are more likely to be taking prescription drugs, which may interact with misused substances. They may also overuse prescription or over-the-counter (OTC) drugs and become dependent on them.
- Older people are more vulnerable to, and vulnerable from, falls when intoxicated.
- They are often more vulnerable to exploitation by others who supply them substances or make them obtain prescription medicines for 'street' use (Wadd et al., 2011).
- Late-onset problem use may also be triggered by life events. Typical triggers have been found to be bereavement, retirement, loneliness, being a carer or having chronic pain (Wadd et al., 2011).

What can we do to address substance misuse in older people?

Screening and brief interventions

Screening for alcohol and drug use is a recommended frontline health promotion strategy for all health and social care workers (NICE, 2010). However, general screening tools for alcohol or drug use are not designed for older people. It can be just as effective to ask directly about drug or alcohol use and what negative effects it may have on the person (i.e. falls, confusion, incontinence, poor sleep). It is likely that older people will experience more shame associated with their substance misuse so it can be difficult for professionals to broach the subject. However, if nobody asks the questions, their problem use may go unnoticed and untreated even longer (see Box 37.1).

Some older people may have dementia or other cognitive impairments, so will not be able to give an accurate history of their substance use. It may help to talk to family or carers, or to assess their substance use in the home environment where there may be clues to their actual behaviour (Drugscope, 2014).

Brief intervention can be delivered to people who are not clearly dependent but may be endangering their health with their drug or alcohol use. Brief intervention is a short, non-confrontational structured conversation that aims to explore with the person their knowledge of the risks involved in the substance. The approach should be to ask open questions about how much the person knows about their substance use and give supportive advice to empower them to consider reducing their use (NHS Health Scotland, 2015). Guidance in delivering brief intervention for alcohol use is recommended for staff in NHS-commissioned services (NICE, 2010).

When to screen or further assess (Figure 37.1)

There should be concern for an older person if they exhibit certain physical symptoms including: frequent falls and injuries, tremor and instability, memory loss and confusion, self neglect, gastrointestinal and liver abnormalities, malnutrition, nausea or changes in eating habits (Royal College of Psychiatrists, 2011). Any of these should prompt basic screening, while evidence of harmful use or dependency is cause for further assessment or referral to specialist services (Wadd et al., 2011).

References

Ayres, R., Eveson, L., Ingram, J. and Telfer, M. (2012) Treatment experience and needs of older drug users in Bristol, UK. *Journal of Substance Use* 17(1): 19–31.

Drugscope (2014) It's about time: Tackling substance misuse in older people. Drugscope and Recovery Partnership.

National Treatment Agency (2011) Addiction to medicine: An investigation into the configuration and commissioning of treatment services to support those who develop problems with prescription-only or over-the-counter medicine. Available at: http://www.nta.nhs.uk/uploads/addictiontomedicinesmay2011a.pdf (accessed 4 October 2017).

NHS Health Scotland (2015) Delivering an ABI: Process, screening tools and guidance notes. NHS Scotland, Edinburgh.

NICE (2010) Alcohol-use disorders: preventing the development of hazardous and harmful drinking. NICE public health guidance 24. London: National Institute for Health and Clinical Excellence.

Public Health England (2013) Drug treatment in England 2012-13. Public Health England.

Royal College of Psychiatrists (2011) Our invisible addicts: First report of the Older Persons' Substance Misuse Working Group of the Royal College of Psychiatrists. London: Royal College of Psychiatrists. Available at: http://www.rcpsych.ac.uk/files/pdf-version/cr165.pdf (accessed 25 September 2017).

Wadd, S., Lapworth, K., Sullivan, M., Forrester, D. and Galvani, S. (2011) Working with older drinkers. Tilda Goldberg Centre, University of Bedfordshire. Available at: http://alcoholresearchuk.org/downloads/finalReports/FinalReport_0085 (accessed 25 September 2017).

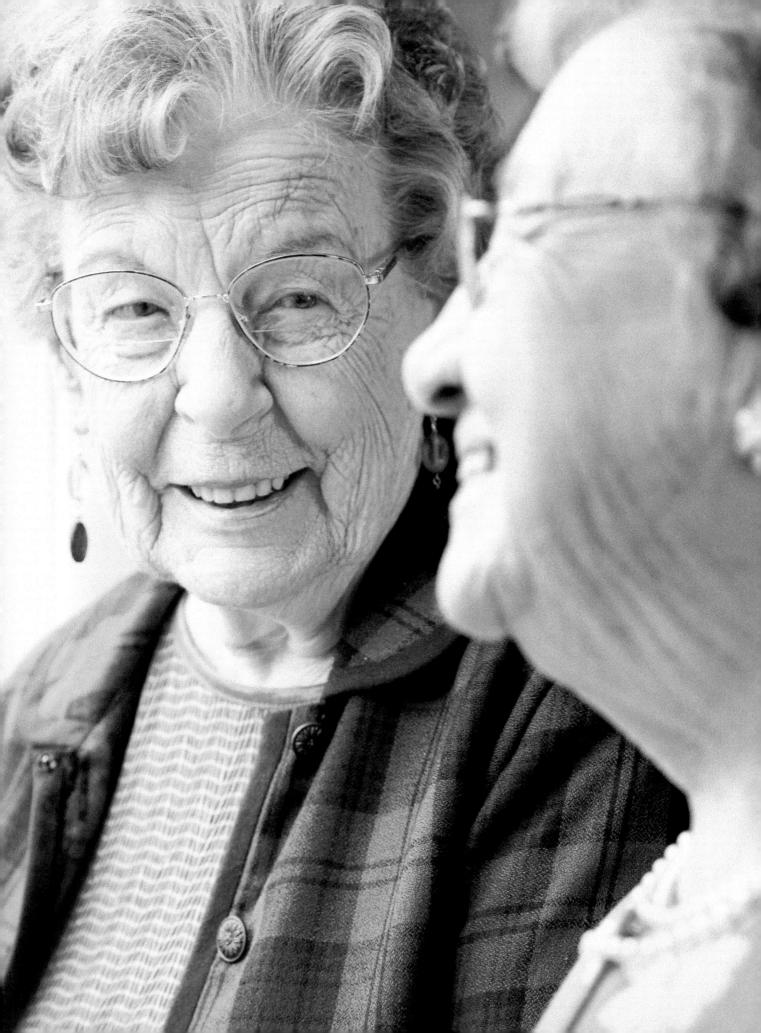

Environments of care and practice

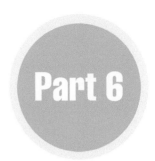

Part 6

Chapters

38 Autonomy and independence

Figure 38.1 A two-dimensional model of independence. Source: Secker *et al.* (2003). Reproduced with permission of Cambridge University Press.

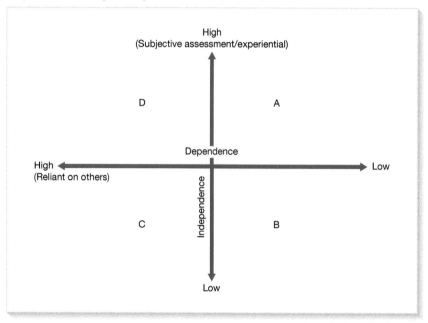

Box 38.1 Case study.

Joan and Norman have been married for 60 years. They live together in their family home, in a quiet suburban street. They have two adult children. Jane, the eldest sibling, lives locally. She has two school-age children, and she works full-time at the local supermarket. Peter, the younger sibling, is also married, and lives a three-hour drive away from his parental home. Norman recently fell, fracturing his hip. After hospitalisation, he has returned to the family home. Joan is helping him with hygiene and toileting needs as he is 'less steady on his feet' than previously. The district nurse has called to take a routine blood sample. While the nurse is there, Jane arrives at the home. Jane takes the District Nurse to one side, and expresses concerns about Joan's continuing ability to cope with Norman's physical care needs. Jane feels that Norman's care needs can no longer be met by Joan. Neither Joan nor Norman have expressed any concerns; however, Joan appears tired and short-tempered. Jane is keen for them to agree to receive regular care visits in order to help both Joan and Norman.

Nursing Older People at a Glance, First Edition. Edited by Josie Tetley, Nigel Cox, Kirsten Jack and Gary Witham.
© 2018 John Wiley & Sons, Ltd. Published 2018 by John Wiley & Sons, Ltd.

People in the UK are living longer, with a life expectancy of approximately 21 years for women and 19 years for men, at the age of 65 (Office for National Statistics, 2015); numbers of those aged over 85 are projected to increase in the next two decades, creating additional demand upon health and social care services (Age UK, 2017). Therefore encouraging older people to live independently might be considered important, and for some older people successful ageing is linked to the ability to maintain one's independence (Smith *et al.*, 2007). If people are able to cope unaided then this places less of a burden on others (Leece and Peace, 2010). However, older people tend to have a more flexible notion of independence, which can change over time.

Secker *et al.* (2003) propose a two-dimensional model that defines dependence as the extent to which we rely on others, or the resources provided for us (Figure 38.1). However, independence is viewed as a subjective state that might differ depending on who we are and the way we feel. It is described as:

> *…the individual's subjective assessment of whether their lived experience matches up to the desired level of choice, social usefulness and autonomy, which in turn depends on their psychological make-up, biography, social context and cultural heritage*
>
> Secker, *et al.*, 2003, p. 380

This definition encourages us to view independence as a personal and highly subjective state, not merely how much we rely on others.

Following the model and case study (Box 38.1), Norman might consider that he is living independently, as he has matched his expectations to his decreased mobility. However, to others he might be perceived as being dependent on Joan. Jane believes that Norman cannot be cared for by Joan any longer, although to Norman, on a subjective level, he is living independently. Norman might place himself in quadrant D of Figure 38.1; he feels independent even though he relies on others. However, Jane might place him in quadrant C – a low level of independence and high dependence on others. Assessing Norman's view of his independence is very important for the nurse when considering care delivery and management.

Respecting autonomy, independence and choice with the needs of older carers

In such situations it is important that nurses can recognise and distinguish between what a patient *wants* (for instance, to be clean and comfortable), and their nursing *needs* (which will be assessed by the nurse in collaboration with the patient, their primary carers and others in the multidisciplinary team), and the *choices* that are available to them.

In the case study, Norman wishes to continue to receive care from Joan in their home. Norman is having his *wants* met, and although he is not as mobile as he would like to be, he nonetheless feels that he is living independently. This situation allows him to exercise choice and self-determination. However, are Norman's *needs* being met?

Assessing Norman's needs is different from what Norman wants. The nurse has a duty to assess his needs (for instance, his mobility and toileting needs) and intervene to support his well-being, but must do so whilst respecting his autonomy. However, although Norman's capacity for self-determination is unchanged, his independence depends upon Joan's well-being.

How the nurse assesses this situation is very important. The nurse must make a holistic assessment, which in this situation means taking into account an older person's social and psychological needs, recognising and respecting their preferences (NMC, 2015), and remaining mindful of their legal duty, under the Human Rights Act 1998, to respect private and family life.

For Norman, part of the nurse's assessment will therefore also require the nurse to consider the changing nature of his family relationships as he (and Joan) are becoming frailer. This is important because their adult children also find themselves with new responsibilities beyond the parental home.

Norman retains his independence only *with* Joan's support. Jane has indicated that Joan may be becoming frail. The nurse takes this into account in the assessment. Although Norman wants Joan to continue to care for him, a nursing assessment may indicate that Joan may not be able to *sustain* her care delivery in a way that is *safe* for *both of them*.

This situation may constitute *an unacceptable risk*. Although providing *choices* is desirable, nurses also need to recognise a person in their care may sometimes make choices that are at odds with professional advice. Therefore, it is essential for nurses to consider not only the patient's autonomy, but also assess risks to others and escalate any concerns according to statutory guidelines or local policy.

References

Age UK (2017) The Health and Care of Older People in England 2017. Available at: https://www.ageuk.org.uk/Documents/EN-GB/For-professionals/Research/The_Health_and_Care_of_Older_People_in_England_2017.pdf (accessed 4 October 2017).

Leece, J. and Peace, S. (2010) Developing new understandings of independence and autonomy in the personalised relationship. *British Journal of Social Work* 40: 1847–1865.

NMC (2015) The Code. London: Nursing and Midwifery Council. Available at: https://www.nmc.org.uk/standards/code/ (accessed 4 October 2017).

Office for National Statistics (2015) Life expectancy at birth and at age 65 for local areas in England and Wales, 2012–14. Newport: Office for National Statistics. Available at: https://www.ons.gov.uk/people-populationandcommunity/birthsdeathsandmarriages/lifeexpectancies (accessed 4 October 2017).

Secker, J., Hill, R., Villeneau, L. and Parkman, S. (2003) Promoting independence: but promoting what and how? *Ageing and Society* 23(3): 375–391.

Smith, J.A., Braunack-Mayer, A., Wittert, G. and Warin, M. (2007) "I've been independent for so damn long!": Independence, masculinity and aging in a help seeking context. *Journal of Aging Studies* 21: 325–335.

39 Transitions in care

Figure 39.1 Older People Acute Care Model (OPAC). Source: Peek *et al.* (2007). Reproduced with permission of Taylor & Francis.

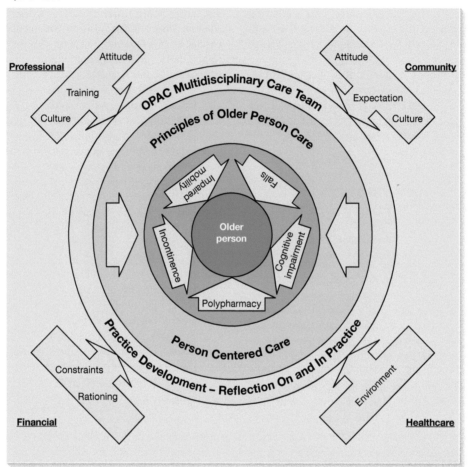

Box 39.1 Best Practice for Older People statements.
Source: Adapted from Bridges *et al.* (2009).

- Maintaining identity: see who I am.
- Creating communities: connect with me.
- Sharing decision-making: involve me.
- Caring for people with mental health needs.
- Caring for people with palliative care needs.
- Caring for people at end of life.
- Meeting needs of nutrition and hydration.
- Promoting continence.
- Promoting mobility and preventing falls.
- Preventing and managing pressure ulcers.

Nursing Older People at a Glance, First Edition. Edited by Josie Tetley, Nigel Cox, Kirsten Jack and Gary Witham.
© 2018 John Wiley & Sons, Ltd. Published 2018 by John Wiley & Sons, Ltd.

Transition into acute care

Transfer to hospital, be it a planned or emergency admission, can have a negative impact on the overall health and well-being of older people. The transition from independent living to a role that requires assistance from healthcare professionals can also fall into the category of unpredictable–involuntary transition (Liddle *et al.*, 2004).

All individuals experience transition in different ways; some become very unsettled whilst others are much more resilient in dealing with life changes. Admission to acute care and the need for healthcare support can also cause individuals to feel defenceless, fearful and worthless, along with a lack of autonomy and control. Alongside this, individuals can feel a reduction in their quality of life and have a reduced ability to engage in meaningful activity (Irvine, 2008). Given the complexity of transitions into acute care settings, treating all older people in the same way has to be challenged. Thus the nurse must understand each older person's experience of transition in order to deliver person-centred care, rather than focusing narrowly on treatment and technical aspects.

Support in acute care environments

Nursing and Midwifery Council (2009) requirements address the vision for best practice in acute care of older people. Based on this guidance, Bridges *et al.* (2009) make suggestions for Best Practice for Older People (BPOP) in acute care (Box 39.1). Fundamental to these guidelines is the notion of nurses moving away from the focus on technical competence to that of broad humanistic caring practice that encompasses person-centred/relationship-centred nursing Many models of person-centred care exist but one has been developed specifically for older person acute care (Peek *et al.*, 2007; see Figure 39.1). The model developed by Peek *et al.* is particularly relevant in the context of this book as it illustrates how many of the issues raised come together and impact on the experiences of an older person in an acute care setting.

In order to develop both person-centred care and relationship-centred care that can promote the importance and centrality of the person and recognise the criticality of interdependence, there are three broad areas that affect transition into and out of acute care environments: respect, decision-making, and choice and communication.

- **Respect:** Care that does not show respect, and which dehumanises and objectifies the older person. Older people perceive ageism, and power relationships still exist in acute care environments, contributing to a lack of respect which threatens sense of identity and involvement (Irvine, 2008).

- **Decision-making and choice:** When assisting transition to acute care, recognise that not all individuals want to participate in the process. This might depend on their level of ill-health, personality and feelings of dependency. Critical to decision-making is that the person has relevant and appropriate information on which to base their decision (Bridges *et al.*, 2009).
- **Communication:** Can help create connections between individuals and significantly affects transition. Poor communication skills cause older people to feel unvalued and unimportant. Staff who listen and plan care around older people's individual needs rather than delivering routinised care, enable older people to feel more in control, leading to a positive experience (McCormack *et al.*, 2008).

Nursing older people in an acute setting is a highly skilled and complex activity that can be assisted by using person-centred approaches to gain understanding and knowledge of each individual.

Conclusion

Older people with acute care needs are likely to have complex needs. Transitions into a different environment can be upsetting and disturbing for an older person. Individuals will vary in their ability to adjust to a transition in care setting. Effective transitions can be enabled through supportive communication, shared decision-making and treating older people with respect.

References

Bridges, J., Flatley, M. and Meyer, J. (2009) Guidance on best practice in acute care. *Nursing Older People* 21(10): 18–20.

Irvine, L.M.C. (2008) Understanding the experience of older people in acute health care. Unpublished PhD thesis, Edinburgh Queen Margaret University.

Liddle, J., Carlson, G. and McKenna, H. (2004) Using a matrix in life transition research. *Qualitative Health Research* 14: 1396–1417.

McCormack, B., Mitchell, E.A., Cook, G., Reed, J. and Childs, S. (2008) Older persons' experiences of whole systems: the impact of health and social care organizational structures. *Journal of Nursing Management* 16(2): 105–114.

Nursing and Midwifery Council (2009) *Guidance for the Care of Older People*. London: NMC.

Peek, C., Higgins, I., Milson-Hawke, S., McMillan, M. and Harper, D. (2007) Towards innovation: The development of a person-centred model of care for older people in acute care. *Contemporary Nurse* 26(2): 164–179.

40 Coordinating care

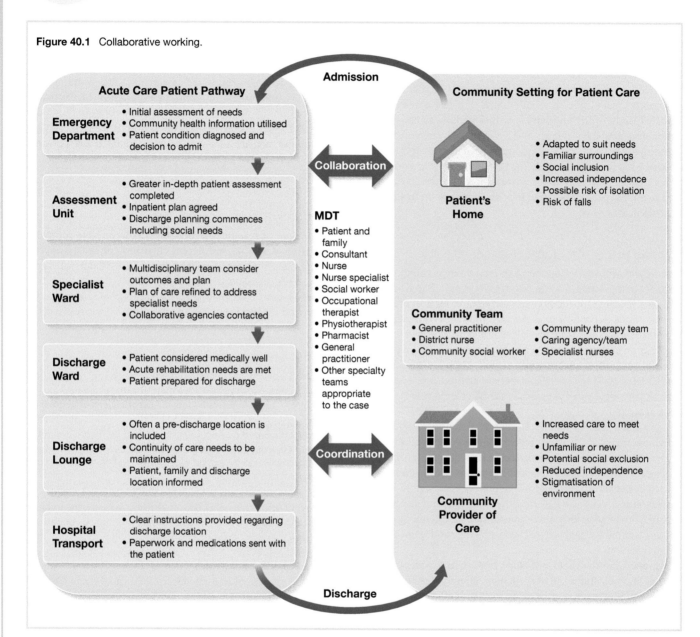

Figure 40.1 Collaborative working.

Complex needs of older people under our care

An older person's needs in both the community and hospital setting are complex and diverse due to many patients having multiple physical illnesses and often having additional requirements to address their functional and mental health needs (Goldberg *et al.*, 2014). Addressing these diverse needs requires a balancing of professional and ethical dilemmas when considering strategies to minimise patient risk whilst still respecting patient autonomy (Janssen *et al.*, 2015). It is therefore understandable how an episode of acute illness requiring hospital admission would further exacerbate the complex needs of an older person. Coupling an acute care setting with the care requirements of older people requires a multidisciplinary team (MDT) approach to coordinate care (Goldberg *et al.*, 2014), which is in line with the project outlined by the Care Quality Commission (CQC) (2015) 'Integrated care for older people: Shaping a health and care system that is designed around the individual'. This directive by the CQC specifically focuses on the complex needs of older people and the need to integrate health and social care services through coordination of different organisations. Arguably the effectiveness of the MDT is imperative to coordinate services, which reduces the risk of the patient pathway becoming fragmented (Care Quality Commission, 2015). Any gap in the continuity of care has an impact on older people, and nurses should provide care that

Nursing Older People at a Glance, First Edition. Edited by Josie Tetley, Nigel Cox, Kirsten Jack and Gary Witham.
© 2018 John Wiley & Sons, Ltd. Published 2018 by John Wiley & Sons, Ltd.

prioritises individual needs but in so doing work in partnership (Nursing and Midwifery Council, 2015). Coordinating care through partnership working will remove possible barriers in order to deliver person-centred care, which is facilitated through an effectively functioning intra- and inter-organisational MDT (Janssen *et al.*, 2015). If there is a gap in service continuity for older people, there is a need to consider how nursing staff can coordinate care more effectively.

Coordinating acute hospital care and discharge planning (Figure 40.1)

The discharge of older people from acute care to the community is complex, which can cause delays. These delays in the discharge process can result in hospital beds being occupied by patients who are deemed medically well; however, due to a patient awaiting continuing care arrangements/agreements the patient cannot be safely discharged from hospital. This is because hospital and community healthcare delivered by the National Health Service is free of charge at the point of delivery, whereas the social care system requires assessment of patient need ahead of agreeing any subsidies to be provided towards the cost of community social care. To coordinate the safe and appropriate discharge of an older person it is important to commence the discharge planning process at the earliest opportunity and not wait until a decision is made that the person is medically well enough to be discharged. This should be the output from the holistic nursing assessment carried out at the point of admission to acute care where social, psychological, emotional and spiritual needs are identified along with the patient's physical health. The nursing role within this process should be to provide a detailed holistic assessment, which focuses on the needs of the individual including their opinions and beliefs. This vital information then allows the nurse to coordinate care with the relevant professionals from within the organisation and liaise with professional representatives from partner organisations, for example social services.

Coordination and nursing ability to provide advocacy for the patient requires nurses to demonstrate effective leadership skills and attributes (Marquis and Huston, 2006). The importance of leadership within the nursing role when caring for older people needs to be further emphasised when considering patients' expectations and their recognition of the nurse role within their care. Effective nursing leadership is therefore imperative in generating a collaborative team, one that is working towards the best possible outcome for the patient.

What is the nursing role within the MDT when coordinating the care of older people?

As identified, the needs of older persons are complex, requiring developed skills by nursing staff to coordinate the delivery of services. Following an older person being admitted to hospital, there is often a transitional phase where increased dependency of care is experienced, resulting in the patient, family and MDT having to make challenging decisions regarding further care environments after discharge (Goldberg *et al.*, 2014). Based on increased patient dependency the coordination of care is likely to include multiple health and social care organisations; therefore the nurse accountable for the delivery of care to the patient must have an understanding of how the services are instigated through correct liaison and communication with relevant representatives from the organisations. For example, if an older person is admitted to hospital and is unable to return home this would require substantial coordination of care through assessing, planning, implementation and evaluation of the care planning process. The nurse coordinating the care for the person will have detailed knowledge and understanding from the assessment, which needs to be utilised when representing the patient's wishes, beliefs and opinions when the MDT meets to discuss the patient case. The nursing role as patient advocate is important as the MDT will often experience situations where the team members will need to deliberate and reflect upon ethical dilemmas relating to interventional strategies that would be appropriate for the individual (Janssen *et al.*, 2015). The nurse, with their in-depth knowledge of the patient, should be central to this discussion, and in a position to coordinate and implement the plan of care, demonstrating the important role of the nurse and their leadership within the MDT.

Conclusion

Assessment of older people should include a full holistic approach, and assessments carried out upon admission to an acute care setting should inform the discharge planning process.

The nurse accountable for the care of the patient should act as the patient's advocate, and a team approach should be developed by collaborative working of intra- and inter-organisational professionals. Effective nursing leadership is imperative to ensure care is coordinated to meet individual patient needs.

References

Care Quality Commission (2015) Integrated care for older people: Shaping a health and care system that is designed around the individual. London: CQC.

Goldberg, S., Cooper, J. and Russell, C. (2014) Developing advanced nursing skills for frail older people. *Nursing Older People* 26(26): 20–23.

Janssen, B.M., Snoeren, M.W.C., Regenmortel, T.V. and Abma, T.A. (2015) Working towards integrated community care for older people: Empowering organisational features from a professional perspective. *Health Policy* 119: 1–8.

Marquis, B.L. and Huston, C.J. (2006) *Leadership roles and Management Functions in Nursing: Theory and Application*. Philadelphia: Lippincott Williams & Wilkins.

Nursing and Midwifery Council (2015) *The Code: Professional standards of practice and behaviour for nurses and midwives*. London: NMC.

41 Care at home

Figure 41.1 Key factors for consideration when providing nursing in the home.

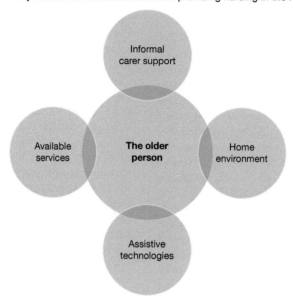

Figure 41.2 The House of Care. Source: https://www.england.nhs.uk/house-of-care/ (accessed July 2017). Contains public sector information licensed under the Open Government Licence v3.0.

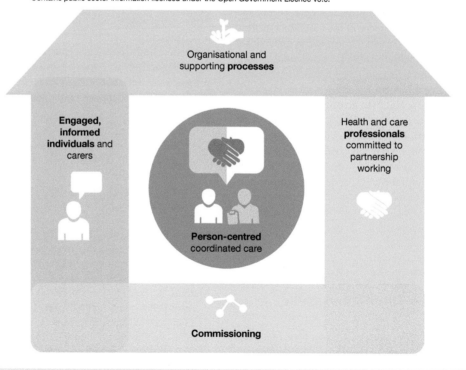

Introduction

In an age where older people are frequently portrayed as a burden on NHS services, it is important to remember that most live active, fulfilling lives and continue to contribute to society. However, as people age, many develop health conditions requiring professional interventions. The political drive for moving healthcare closer to home (Monitor, 2015; NHS England et al., 2014) has resulted in an increasing number of patients who would previously have been cared for in hospital, receiving support and sophisticated clinical interventions within the home environment (Department of Health, 2014; The Queen's Nursing Institute, 2012). The provision of such care within non-clinical environments provides diverse challenges for community nurses, particularly those working with older people – the latter are likely to have complex health and social care needs.

Integrated healthcare

The provision of high-quality care in the home relies on multi-disciplinary working aligned with the concept of integrated care, which emphasises the centrality of the patient's experience and requires the orchestration of services to avoid duplication and fragmentation of care (Figure 41.1). The 'House of Care' model (Figure 41.2) is a concept aimed at achieving this for people with long-term conditions, 80% of whom are aged 65 and over (Coulter et al., 2013). The house is built around personalised care planning and is underpinned by local commissioning. The roof represents the organisational systems required for the implementation of efficient care processes, and the walls represent patients, carers and professionals who work in partnership to achieve mutually determined goals that develop, support and utilise the patient's potential for self-care.

Nursing in the home

A range of community nursing services provide care and support for older people in their homes. The largest and longest established is district nursing, which can be traced back to the 1800s (Queen's Nursing Institute, 2012). Older people account for the largest proportion of District Nurses' caseloads, and one in four people aged 75 and over require district nursing interventions, a figure that rises to one in two for people aged over 85 years (Queen's Nursing Institute, 2012). District Nurses work with some of the most vulnerable people in society as, in addition to having multiple diagnoses and polypharmacy, many are frail, housebound and dependent on others (Queen's Nursing Institute, 2012). As well as providing the clinical care that patients require, District Nurses play a pivotal role in the coordination of multidisciplinary care delivery and have a responsibility to support independence and improve and protect health (Department of Health, 2014).

Home health assessments

A thorough patient assessment is essential in any context. Within a person's home, this includes assessment of the environment in terms of its suitability for home nursing and safe living. Current statistics show that 61% of people aged 65 and over own their home (Department for Communities and Local Government, 2015). However, 67% of this group are living in poverty, and one in five of all homes occupied by older people fail the decent homes standard (Age UK, 2016). Community nurses can facilitate referrals to sources of help, but improvements and adaptations may take considerable time to be actioned. Providing care in poor environments can be hazardous to both nurses and patients, and full risk assessments are vital. A non-judgemental stance is essential and, if compromises have to be agreed, discussions should be sensitively handled in order to maintain patient dignity.

Carer support

Even with the best available care packages, many older people could not remain at home without the support of informal carers. In 2014, around one in six of the population in England was providing informal care for an older person, and the number of older carers is rapidly increasing (Carers UK, 2016); thus, the proportion of carers who are also in poor health is also likely to increase. Hence, it is important for community nurses and other healthcare professionals to consider the health needs of carers along with those of the patient.

References

Age UK (2016) Later Life in the United Kingdom. Available at: http://www.ageuk.org.uk/Documents/EN-GB/Factsheets/Later_Life_UK_factsheet.pdf?dtrk=true (accessed 26 September 2017).

Carers UK (2016) State of caring 2016. Available at: http://www.carersuk.org/for-professionals/policy/policy-library/state-of-caring-2016 (accessed 26 September 2017).

Coulter, A., Roberts, S. and Dixon, A. (2013) Delivering better services for people with long-term conditions: Building the house of care. London: King's Fund.

Department for Communities and Local Government (2015) English Housing Survey Headline Report 2014-15. Available at: https://www.gov.uk/government/uploads/system/uploads/attachment_data/file/501065/EHS_Headline_report_2014-15.pdf (accessed 26 September 2017).

Department of Health (2014) Transforming primary care. Available at: https://www.gov.uk/government/uploads/system/uploads/attachment_data/file/304139/Transforming_primary_care.pdf (accessed 26 September 2017).

Monitor (2015) Moving healthcare closer to home: Summary. Available at: https://www.gov.uk/government/uploads/system/uploads/attachment_data/file/459400/moving_healthcare_closer_to_home_summary.pdf (accessed 26 September 2017).

NHS England, Care Quality Commission, Health Education England, Monitor, Public Health England and Trust Development Authority (2014) NHS five year forward view. London: NHS England.

Queen's Nursing Institute (2012) Nursing people at home. Available at: https://www.qni.org.uk/resources/nursing-people-home-report (accessed 26 September 2017).

42 Social isolation and loneliness

Figure 42.1 Factors that impact on social isolation.

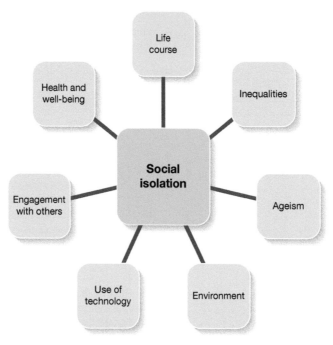

Table 42.1 Understanding loneliness and social isolation. Source: Adapted from Davidson and Rossall (2014).

Loneliness	Social isolation
Can be understood as an individual's personal, subjective sense of lacking desired affection, closeness, and social interaction with others Although loneliness has a social aspect, it is also defined by an individual's subjective emotional state. Loneliness is more dependent on the quality than the number of relationships	Is a lack of contact with family or friends, community involvement, or access to services

Nursing Older People at a Glance, First Edition. Edited by Josie Tetley, Nigel Cox, Kirsten Jack and Gary Witham.
© 2018 John Wiley & Sons, Ltd. Published 2018 by John Wiley & Sons, Ltd.

Our social engagement and relationships with others are important to our physical, emotional and psychosocial well-being. Understanding this is important. An evidence review on loneliness identified that over one million older people say that they often or always feel lonely, and 49% of people aged 65 in the UK report that the television or pets are their main form of company (Davidson and Rossall, 2014). For older people, research has identified that being socially isolated and lonely was associated with increased death rates (Steptoe *et al.*, 2013). It has also been argued that being lonely and socially isolated is as damaging to health as smoking 15 cigarettes a day (Holt-Lunstad *et al.*, 2015). While social isolation and loneliness are often referred to together it is important to recognise that these are different but related concepts. The distinctions between loneliness and social isolation have been identified in an Age UK report on loneliness (Table 42.1).

Older people are, however, at increased risk of being socially isolated for a range of interrelated factors (Figure 42.1). This chapter will look at ways in which nurses can help older people to be more socially connected in ways that can positively impact on their health and well-being.

The impact of any physical health conditions can contribute to situations where people feel more socially isolated. In particular, any long-term condition that reduces mobility can restrict access to the external environment and lead to a more sedentary lifestyle. Inequalities related to a range of factors such as lack of money, lack of resources or discrimination based on gender, sexuality or ethnicity can also contribute to older people being at increased risk of social isolation or loneliness. Ageism is particularly important when considering what interventions might help reduce social isolation as incorrect assumptions can often be made about the interests and capacities of older people, particularly when it comes to new innovations in society. Life-course, events and relationships in people's lives can also lead to some older people being more at risk of being socially isolated and lonely than others. In terms of connections with others, divorce, death of a partner, adult children living at a distance, lack of support for family carers or difficult family relationships may then all increase the risk of social isolation.

In tackling social isolation and loneliness it is important to start with the individual to assess their circumstances to understand if they are lonely or socially isolated and what the reasons are for this. In addition, their interests impact on what type of intervention or activity could suit them.

There are many national and local interventions that can support people to age in place. This is important as living in a familiar environment can help older people maintain independent living in the community and decrease the risk of social isolation. One way of helping people overcome social isolation is the promotion of physical and social activities outside of the home; these do not have to be expensive. A range of examples that a nurse might want to consider signposting an older person to are:

- **Local walking clubs:** Walking is an accessible activity that also has health benefits, such as weight management, management of blood pressure and balance, and it can help with connections to the community.
- **Social eating clubs:** These might be organised luncheon clubs in local community centres or community developed social eating opportunities in public places that provide access to affordable food in a sociable space. Initiatives such as these can have additional health benefits for people who live alone as shopping and cooking fresh food for one person can be difficult to maintain on a regular basis. However, older adults with tremors or swallowing difficulties might be uncomfortable eating socially.
- **Men in Sheds:** Taking account of different gender needs for participation in meaningful activities, charities such as Age UK have supported 'Men in Sheds' as an initiative to support older men who want the company of others to share and learn new skills. The space and paid support are provided by Age UK but the participant 'Shedders' choose the activities. Typical activities include woodworking, intergenerational skill-sharing, and socialising.
- **Befriending/listening services:** There are many local and national organisations that link lonely or socially isolated older people with volunteers for social interaction. These vary locally but include, for example, Age UK, the British Red Cross, Alzheimer's Society and the Royal Voluntary Service. Some of these support social engagement in the person's home, others are focused on helping the older person to get out of their home to meet others, or maintain engagement with activities. There are also telephone-based befriending services, which might suit some older adults.
- **Peer to peer technology support:** Although older people have seen many technological developments in their lifetime their engagement with new and emerging technologies is more limited. Participatory work with older people across Europe found that peer-to-peer approaches to learning that used play and creative learning gave older people increased opportunities for and greater confidence about engaging with new technologies via the internet such as Skype, tablet technologies and to a lesser degree social media (Tetley *et al.*, 2015). Being able to engage with internet-based systems is particularly important as public and private services are increasingly moving online, which further increases the risk of social isolation and social exclusion for older people.

Nurses are in a unique place to assess the social needs of older people alongside their health needs. Being aware of simple and creative opportunities for community engagement that can support their clients' physical, mental and social needs can then improve health outcomes for older people.

References

Davidson, S. and Rossall, P. (2014) Age UK Loneliness Evidence Review. London: Age UK.

Holt-Lunstad, J., Smith, T.B., Baker, M., Harris, T. and Stephenson, D. (2015) Loneliness and social isolation as risk factors for mortality: a meta-analytic review. *Perspectives on Psychological Science* 10: 227–237.

Steptoe, A., Shankar, A., Demakakos, P. and Wardle, J. (2013) Social isolation, loneliness, and all-cause mortality in older men and women. *Proceedings of the National Academy of Sciences* 110: 5797–5801.

Tetley, J., Holland, C., Waights, V., Hughes, J., Holland, S. and Warren, S, (2015) Exploring new technologies through playful peer-to-peer engagement in informal learning. In: Prendergast D. and Garattini C. (eds), *Aging and the Digital Life Course*. New York/Oxford: Berghahn, pp. 39–62.

43 Communal living

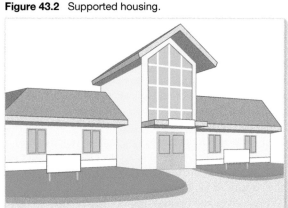

Figure 43.1 Almshouse.

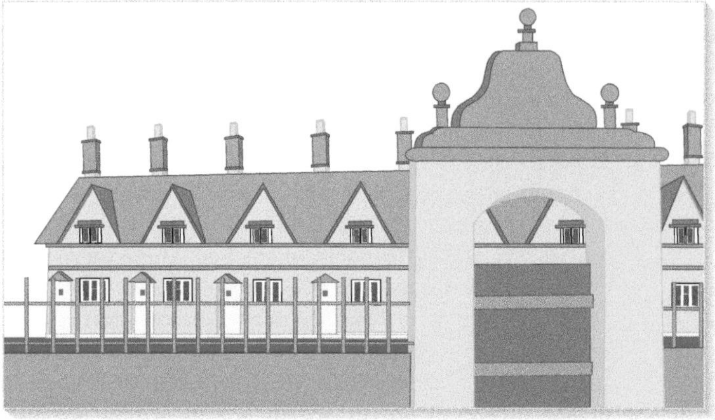

Figure 43.2 Supported housing.

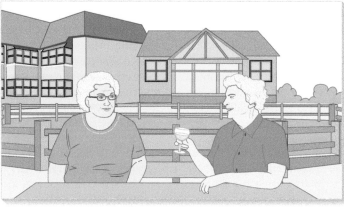

Figure 43.3 Communal setting.

Nursing Older People at a Glance, First Edition. Edited by Josie Tetley, Nigel Cox, Kirsten Jack and Gary Witham.
© 2018 John Wiley & Sons, Ltd. Published 2018 by John Wiley & Sons, Ltd.

The vast majority of older people in the UK (and in many other countries, too) remain living in non-specialist accommodation in age-mixed communities – either in homes where they may have lived for a good while, or in smaller houses or apartments where they have 'downsized' for convenience. However, a smaller proportion of older people move into grouped living arrangements, with or without care services, and involving different kinds of social arrangements (Rowles and Bernard, 2013). It is important for nurses to have some understanding of these different kinds of arrangements, which can have an impact on how older patients are supported in the community.

Almshouses

One of the earliest forms of specialised accommodation designed for the needs of older people was the traditional almshouse, still to be seen dotted around the country, often as small groups of attractive old cottages gathered around a garden or courtyard.

Almshouses have been recorded in Britain from the tenth century (Figure 43.1). The oldest that still exists today is the Hospital of St Cross in Winchester, dating from 1132. Almshouses are essentially charitable institutions run by charities or trustees, who select the residents based on their own criteria. They are generally aimed at older men or women, often targeted at poorer members of the community, and sometimes at local people or people who had followed a particular trade or occupation. Residents do not have security of tenure, but almshouses are considered to be homes for life provided the resident can continue to live independently. Nurses can play a crucial role in enabling these residents to maintain their independence and keep their homes.

Social housing for older people

When the connections began to be made between public health and the provision of adequate housing for all, local authorities and subsequently housing associations and trusts became involved in providing 'social' housing. The idea of specialist housing for older people also spread more widely, with the development of small self-contained homes for rent. These might be small flats or bungalows, again often grouped together in local communities like the almshouses, regarded as suitable for the needs of single older people or couples. Many of these kinds of accommodation now have alarm systems fitted, linked to a central call centre. Residents retain their own GPs.

Sheltered housing

What came next was the development of 'sheltered housing' (Tinker, 2014). This is now sometimes called 'supported housing', which may also be provided for younger adults with special needs; or else 'retirement housing', which reflects an emphasis on independence-with-security (Figure 43.2). Sheltered housing typically has dozens of flats built as a 'scheme', which generally also has a common room area, and possibly a communal kitchen and a guest suite for visitors. Originally most sheltered housing schemes had the services of an on-site warden (manager), but due to budget restrictions this generally gave way to off-site management and the use of alarm systems and telephone checks on residents. Residents have their own GPs and access to health and medical services just as they would if they were living in general housing. While sheltered housing is very often for rent and let to people with few financial resources, there is a parallel market in retirement housing for sale, offering similar arrangements to sheltered housing but more luxurious in terms of fixtures and fittings, and sometimes with larger rooms. Owners are restricted to selling their retirement home to buyers over the required age (e.g. 55+ or 60+).

Retirement villages

There are also various 'retirement villages' for this age group, often located in out-of-town areas with more and larger houses, and many more facilities. The early twenty-first century saw the development of more of these villages as part of a boom in 'extra care housing' – a way of providing for older people's changing needs while avoiding the necessity of a care home admission. This accommodation is designed for accessibility (e.g. doors wide enough for wheelchairs). An extra-care housing scheme is usually large, with anything from dozens to a few hundred apartments, because scale is needed to support the extra facilities on offer. A large extra-care scheme may have on-site a bar, bistro, restaurant, gym, hairdressing salon, computer suite, workshop, craft room and shop. These facilities are aimed at keeping people active and socially involved for as long as possible. However, as the name implies, extra-care housing also intrinsically involves arrangements for care services within the facility. The idea is that as people's needs change (e.g. during a short illness, or when returning after a hospital admission) there is the flexibility to arrange additional temporary support, which can be scaled back as the person improves. While very few employ a nurse directly, there

are often specific arrangements for nursing services alongside other care services and dementia care. Some extra-care schemes have a specialised on-site unit for people living with dementia.

For some people, living in their own home within these communal settlings is seen as the best environment for later years (Figure 43.3), and many extra-care housing schemes have long waiting lists. However, as with any other community, there will always be residents who do not fit in, or don't want to take part in communal activities, and it is possible for individuals to feel lonely even in a thriving scheme. Also, despite the intention that the 'extra care' can provide for people's health needs as they age, severe behavioural problems may be considered too difficult to manage alongside other residents.

Co-housing

What most of these different forms of grouped housing have in common is that residents generally have little say in who lives alongside them, and they may have very little in common except for old age. The exception, perhaps, is in those places (almshouses, some sheltered housing schemes) that are provided for specific groups, for example retired tradespeople such as brewers, seafarers, actors or service personnel; or for people with vision impairments; or for people with particular religious faiths or cultural backgrounds.

Some people do aim more purposefully for a shared life as they age, for example by setting up or joining a co-housing community. Here residents buy or rent their own private property, but share in scheduled communal activities such as shared meals and decision-making meetings. Co-housing, already fairly common in some other countries, is starting to grow in the UK. These communities are often intergenerational but some developments are specifically for older people. Advocates of co-housing say that the long process of community-building while people develop these schemes, and involving applicants in the community while they wait for a vacancy contributes enormously to the success of living together.

Conclusion

So, even though most older people in the UK remain living in 'ordinary' housing, it is useful for nurses to understand something about the various kinds of grouped living for older people. These arrangements are part of the context, as people age, for the maintenance of health, managing of disabilities, and recovery from illness.

References

Rowles, G.D. and Bernard, M. (2013) The meaning and significance of place in old age.In:Rowles, G.D. and Bernard, M. (eds), *Environmental Gerontology: Making Meaningful Places in Old Age*. Springer, pp. 3–24.

Tinker, A. (2014) *Older People in Modern Society*, 4th edn. London: Routledge.

44 Assistive technologies

Box 44.1 Examples of current assistive technologies, telecare, telehealth and mHealth.
Source: Adapted from Dewsbury and Ballard (2012); TSA (2013); and Alzheimer's Society (2015).

Telecare

Equipment to provide care from a distance and support independence and reduce risks, connected through a base unit in a person's home to a monitoring centre.

Equipment that client activates when needing help
- Pendant alarm – worn on neck, wrist or belt.
- Bogus caller button – by the front door.
- Pull cord – built into the home.

Equipment that activates automatically
- Fall detector – equipment that detects a fall (based on impact).
- Environmental sensors – detecting smoke, carbon, gas, flood, extreme temperature.
- Movement sensors – monitor general health, or specific, such as a bed sensor or chair sensor (to detect falls or person getting lost); door exit sensor.

Specific equipment
- Locating technologies, e.g. GPS trackers – for people with dementia or learning disabilities to support independence.
- Medication dispensers.
- Equipment for people with hearing or sight problems – flashing beacon connected to telephone or doorbell and vibrating pillow.

Assistive technology

Equipment to support independence, safety and easier completion of tasks in everyday life. Usually stand-alone.

Equipment for daily living
- Automated prompts and reminders.
- Clocks and calendars.
- Easy-to-use homeware (e.g. cups with two handles, good grip cutlery, non-slip trays).

Equipment for mobility
- Such as walking frames and stairlifts.

Equipment for communication
- Hearing aids, text phone.

Telehealth and telemedicine

Equipment to manage long-term health conditions from a distance.

Examples:
- Blood pressure monitor.
- Pulse oximeter – to monitor oxygen levels in patients with asthma or COPD.
- Glucose meter.
- Body weight scales.

mHealth/mCare

Smart phone applications providing telecare or telehealth support.

Box 44.2 Good practice in using locating technologies with people with dementia to manage wander-walking. Source: Mental Welfare Commission (2015). Reproduced with permission of Mental Welfare Commission for Scotland.

- Consider causes of behaviour.
- Assess the risks to the individual.
- Consider alternatives to use instead of technology.
- Identify if 'wandering technology' is available and appropriate.
- Ascertain views of the resident, relatives and the care team.
- Consider ethical implications, the benefits and disadvantages of the system.
- Consider legal implications for the resident, in particular the possible use of incapacity legislation.
- Formulate individual care plan.
- Ensure staff and relatives understand the care plan.
- Monitor implementation of care plan.
- Review the care plan frequently.

Figure 44.1 Telecare system connecting a telecare client to response centre.

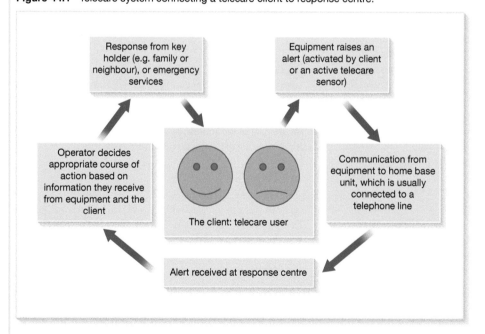

Response from key holder (e.g. family or neighbour), or emergency services

Equipment raises an alert (activated by client or an active telecare sensor)

Operator decides appropriate course of action based on information they receive from equipment and the client

The client: telecare user

Communication from equipment to home base unit, which is usually connected to a telephone line

Alert received at response centre

Nursing Older People at a Glance, First Edition. Edited by Josie Tetley, Nigel Cox, Kirsten Jack and Gary Witham.
© 2018 John Wiley & Sons, Ltd. Published 2018 by John Wiley & Sons, Ltd.

The role of assistive technology to support older people

Assistive technology can support independence of older people in various ways. Telecare belongs under the umbrella term of 'assistive technology', and these two are often referred to as AT/TC. Telecare is care where care receiver and carer are at a distance from each other, using information and communication technology to be contacted, often in an automated way (Figure 44.1) (TSA, 2013). The equipment can help with everyday tasks (such as easy-to-use homeware), support safety and reduce risks (mobility aids, environmental sensors), assist in timely help in case of an accident (telecare system), or support management of long-term health condition (telehealth, medication dispenser) (Box 44.1).

The increased use of assistive technology and telecare stems from various social and technological developments, notably the ageing population and increasing health and social care costs, the lower number of unpaid carers, and the increased aspirations of older people to live independent and active lives.

Benefits of assistive technology and telecare

Telecare can be beneficial for the older person, their unpaid carers and for their care providers. For the older person the equipment can support their independence and living in the community, both by enabling them to do tasks they would otherwise struggle with, keep them safe and delay admission to residential care. For the unpaid carers, many studies refer to the key benefit as increased 'peace of mind' and reduced stress and concern (Jarrold and Yeandle, 2009). In situations when telecare increases the independence of the older person, it can also enhance the independence of the carer, in some cases enabling them to continue working (Jarrold and Yeandle, 2009).

Accessing equipment

The telecare market is fragmented, which can be a challenge for those trying to access equipment. This can be done through social services, when it is based on assessment of needs (although in some areas certain equipment, such as a pendant alarm, is available for everyone over a certain age). Through the NHS, telecare and assistive technology can be a part of a care package to bring older patients home from hospital. Equipment can also be purchased independently, through private sector companies, ageing or disability charities, or through supported housing. Some charities also support certain groups; for example, Blind Veterans provide training and long-term loan of equipment. Trying to navigate the market and choose the right equipment can be challenging. The costs attached to the equipment are also varied: it can be free, have a one-off cost, or a monthly fee. This varies based on the equipment and whether it is equipment that can be used independently by the client or if it requires monitoring and service. The cost of the equipment can create a barrier to accessing it.

Supporting equipment use

As highlighted above, accessing equipment can be a challenge for an older person or their family members. When choosing what equipment and from which provider they will need to balance cost and value for money with understanding if the equipment meets their needs and is easy to use. Further, they need to be able to trust that the equipment does what they think it does, and that they can depend on the equipment.

In the assessment for telecare it is important to understand the everyday life context of the older person. The factors that impact on their equipment use include whether they are living in their own home or in a care home, and if they live alone or with someone. The health conditions of the older person can impact on their equipment use – for example whether they have a physical, cognitive or mental condition or a sensory impairment. Also wider issues can have an impact, such as the individual's needs and abilities, their previous experiences with technology and attitude towards equipment. It is important to note that there is no one typical older person who uses this equipment. Therefore the personalisation of the equipment and understanding the social and everyday life context where the equipment will be used is vital, while remembering that there are situations when telecare is not appropriate (Dewsbury and Ballard, 2012).

Box 44.2 has guidelines on using locating technologies, or wandering technologies, with people with dementia. These guidelines can be adapted in considering the suitability of other technologies.

References

Alzheimer's Society (2015) Assistive technology – devices to help with everyday living. Alzheimer's Society factsheet.

Dewsbury, G. and Ballard D. (2012) Is your home telecare aware? *Nursing and Residential Care* 14(8): 422–424.

Jarrold, K. and Yeandle, S. (2009) 'A weight off my mind': exploring the impact and potential benefits of telecare for unpaid carers in Scotland. Glasgow: Carers Scotland.

Mental Welfare Commission (2005) Safe to Wander? Principles and guidance on good practice in caring for residents with dementia and related disorders where consideration is being given to the use of wandering technologies in care homes and hospitals. Edinburgh: Mental Welfare Commission.

TSA (2013) Telecare and Telehealth: the technology behind the service. Telecare Services Association. http://www.tsa-voice.org.uk/consumer-services/telecare-and-telehealth (accessed 27 September 2017).

45 Older prisoners

Figure 45.1 Change in the age profile of the prison population in England and Wales since 2002. Source: Butler Trust (2015). Reproduced with permission of The Butler Trust.

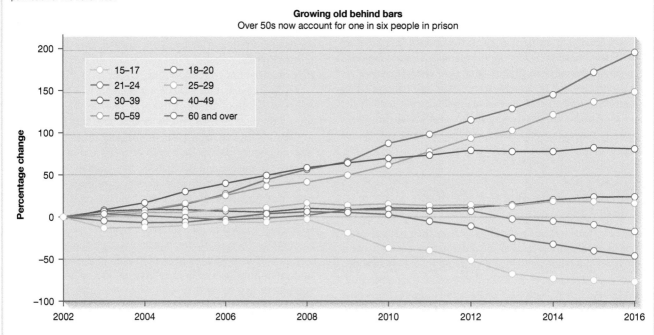

Growing old behind bars
Over 50s now account for one in six people in prison

Figure 45.2 The Older prisoner Health and Social Care Assessment and Plan (OHSCAP). Source: Senior *et al.* (2013).

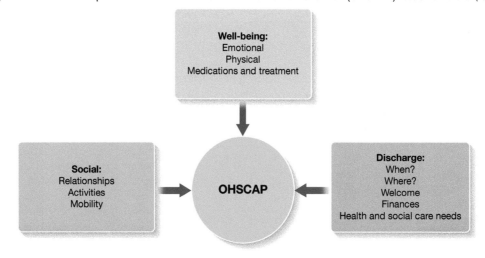

Well-being:
Emotional
Physical
Medications and treatment

Social:
Relationships
Activities
Mobility

OHSCAP

Discharge:
When?
Where?
Welcome
Finances
Health and social care needs

Box 45.1 Department of Health guidance for release of older prisoners. Source: Senior *et al.* (2013, p.4).

- A health and social care needs assessment history being forwarded by the healthcare team to the offender manager.
- The conduction of a pre-release health and welfare assessment.
- An assessment by a social worker, conducted face-to-face.
- Collaboration with external organisations.
- The organisation of a care package.
- Formal arrangements for loans of occupational therapy equipment.
- A pre-release course specifically for older and retired prisoners.

Nursing Older People at a Glance, First Edition. Edited by Josie Tetley, Nigel Cox, Kirsten Jack and Gary Witham.
© 2018 John Wiley & Sons, Ltd. Published 2018 by John Wiley & Sons, Ltd.

People aged over 60 are the fastest growing age group in the UK prison population, with an increase of 150% between 2002 and 2015 (Figure 45.1). The growing number of older prisoners is not necessarily due to a direct rise in crime in this population; rather, demographic changes, changes in sentencing practices and an increased level of crime reporting have all contributed to this increase. In addition, there has been a rise in people being convicted at an older age for historic offences, with many serving long sentences for sexual offences (Senior *et al.*, 2013).

Health needs

Those entering prisons are often in poorer health than the general population and many have the health characteristics of someone ten years their senior (Senior *et al.*, 2013). However, older prisoners can be reluctant to disclose health problems for fear of stigma or bullying, or due to a more stoic outlook on life. This can lead to their needs being unmet, which can then have a detrimental effect on health. A study undertaken in the Northwest of England (Hayes *et al.*, 2012) suggests that there are high rates of physical disorder, such as osteoarthritis, diabetes and hypertension in the over-50 male prison population, and those in the 50–59-year-old age group were more likely to have a mental illness such as depression.

The environment

The prison environment is problematic for older prisoners, as prisons are not designed for older people; as a result this group are often disadvantaged when compared to younger offenders. Old prison buildings and the physical layout can lead to access problems, especially for those with a disability (Senior *et al.*, 2013). Based on recommendations from NACRO and the Department of Health it is suggested (Senior *et al.*, 2013) that support and care for older people in prison can be made easier by simple adaptations such as:

- making doors and windows open more easily;
- using less harsh lighting;
- having radiators that can be adjusted;
- improved provision of special cutlery, plates, bowls and trays;
- lower television shelves;
- more appropriate seating in cells.

Meeting these needs can, however, be problematic as the prison culture supports a 'one size fits all' approach and prison officers are under pressure to treat all prisoners in the same way (Williams, 2012).

The prison nurse's role

For the nurse, there are also challenges when trying to promote health in the older prison population. However, with that challenge comes an opportunity to provide access to healthcare for people who might not normally come into regular contact with health and social care services. Hence, there are positive opportunities for health education, counselling and treatment, as well as wider levels of screening for infectious diseases on admission to prison (Easley, 2011).

Assessing the needs of older prisoners

The Older prisoner Health and Social Care Assessment and Plan (OHSCAP) assessment process can help prison staff assess the needs of older prisoners; Figure 45.2 gives an overview of this tool. The assessment is divided into three areas: well-being, social care and discharge from prison. The assessment process should take account of information that was provided when the older person was first taken into prison but also take account of any new information that has come to light more recently (Senior *et al.*, 2013). While issues that might impact on the health and well-being of an older person in prison are important, the OHSCAP tool recognises that it is also important to think about the factors that might impact on the person when they are being discharged from prison. The OHSCAP tool can be accessed at https://www.ncbi.nlm.nih.gov/books/NBK259264/.

Older prisoners in the community

Research with older prisoners has identified that they struggle more than younger prisoners with resettlement into the community because they more commonly have reduced social networks and are more likely to be suffering from health and mobility problems (Senior *et al.*, 2013). The same research identified an increased risk of suicide amongst older people who have been in prison, one that needs greater attention and active support both before and after release from prison.

In order for older people to be supported in the community, Senior *et al.* (2013) highlight Department of Health guidance that identifies requirements when planning for the release of older prisoners (Box 45.1).

The community and hospital nurses' role

While the number of older people in the community who have been to prison is still relatively small, it is likely to be an increasing population who will have complex health and social care needs. Nurses will need to work closely with the multidisciplinary team such as social workers, probation officers and housing teams to support effective care in the community. Assessment of mental health needs is particularly important, and support to manage activities of daily living such as cooking, cleaning and laundry, which were previously managed in an institutional setting, needs to be considered.

References

Butler Trust (2015) Management and care of older prisoners. London: The Butler Trust. Available at: http://www.butlertrust.org.uk/management-and-care-of-older-prisoners/ (accessed 6 October 2017).

Easley, C.E. (2011) Together we can make a difference: The case for transnational action for improved health in prisons. *Public Health* 125(10): 675–679.

Hayes, J.A., Burns, A., Turnbull, P. and Shaw, J.J. (2012) The health and social needs of older male prisoners. *International Journal of Geriatric Psychiatry* 27: 1155–1162.

Senior, J., Forsyth, K., Walsh, E., O'Hara, K., Stevenson, C., Hayes, A. et al. (2013) Health and social care services for older male adults in prison: the identification of current service provision and piloting of an assessment and care planning model. *Health Services and Delivery Research* 1(5).

Williams, J. (2012) Social care and older prisoners. *Journal of Social Work* 13(5): 471–491.

Index

Nursing Older People at a Glance, First Edition. Edited by Josie Tetley, Nigel Cox, Kirsten Jack and Gary Witham.
© 2018 John Wiley & Sons, Ltd. Published 2018 by John Wiley & Sons, Ltd.

Notes

Notes

Notes

Notes

Notes